CHRIS PENMAN

99 HACKS FOR HEALTH

Transform Your Health, Enhance Your Energy, Reclaim Your Life

Copyright © 2024 by Chris Penman

©2024 Chris Penman. All rights reserved. No part of this publication may be reproduced, distributed, or transmitted in any form or by any means, including photocopying, recording, or other electronic or mechanical methods, without the prior written permission of the publisher, except in the case of brief quotations embodied in critical reviews and certain other noncommercial uses permitted by copyright law. For permission requests, write to the publisher, addressed "Attention: Permissions Coordinator," at the address below.

CCP PUBLICATIONS

DISCLAIMER: This book is provided for information purposes only and does not constitute medical, legal, or other professional advice. The strategies, tips, and tools contained herein are not intended as a substitute for consulting with a medical professional. All matters regarding your health require medical supervision. The author and publisher disclaim any liability arising directly or indirectly from the use of this material. Any financial claims referenced in this book are illustrative and not guaranteed. Readers are advised to consult a professional before making any major health or financial decisions.

First edition

This book was professionally typeset on Reedsy. Find out more at reedsy.com

Contents

IMPORTANT - READ THIS FIRST   v
INTRODUCTION   x

1 WAKE UP TO WELLNESS   1
  Morning Mastery   1
  Power Breakfasts   4
  Early Bird Exercise   8

2 MENTAL CLARITY THROUGH MINIMALISM   15
  Declutter Your Space   15
  Simplify Your Diet   19
  Streamline Your Thoughts   22

3 BEAT STRESS BEFORE IT BEGINS   29
  Recognize Stress Signals   29
  Quick Stress Relief Techniques   32
  Long-Term Stress Management   35

4 OPTIMISE YOUR SLEEP   42
  Creating a Sleep Sanctuary   42
  Pre-Sleep Rituals   46
  Sleep Schedules   50

5 HYDRATION HACKS   56
  Understanding Hydration   56
  Fun with Fluids   60
  Hydration Monitoring   63

6 MOVEMENT FOR LONGEVITY   69
  Daily Movement Goals   69

Fun Fitness	72
Age-Defying Exercises	76
7 NUTRITION KNOW-HOW	82
Fundamentals of Balanced Eating	82
Superfoods and Their Superpowers	86
Smart Snacking	89
8 MINDFULNESS AND INNER PEACE	95
Basics of Mindfulness	95
Meditation Made Simple	98
Gratitude and Positivity	102
9 BUILDING RESILIENCE	109
Emotional Resilience	109
Physical Resilience	112
Cognitive Resilience	115
10 LIFELONG HABITS FOR HEALTH	122
Routine Building	122
Technology for Health	127
Community and Connection	130
11 SOCIAL WELLNESS AND RELATIONSHIPS	136
Building Strong Connections	136
Family Dynamics and Wellness	140
Social Well-being in the Community	143
EMBRACING YOUR OPTIMAL SELF	151

IMPORTANT - READ THIS FIRST

Hi, I'm Chris Penman, and I'm grateful you took the opportunity to get this book. If you're ready to transform your health, enhance your energy, and reclaim your life, then you're in the right place. This guide is your first step towards a new you.

I've been immersed in the world of holistic health and wellness for over 35 years. Throughout this time, I've realized that despite widespread interest, there remains a host of misconceptions and unanswered questions regarding truly effective, sustainable practices for a healthier life. Compelled by this need for clarity and genuine transformation, I decided to create this book, a compendium of 99 essential hacks to guide you through the missteps and misinformation.

After all, maybe you've tried countless diets that promise miraculous results, only to find yourself back at square one, feeling more disillusioned than ever. The cycle of temporary success followed by inevitable backslide can be frustrating and disheartening.

Maybe you've joined gyms or fitness programs with enthusiasm, believing each time that this would be the change you needed. Yet, despite your best intentions and investments, the initial burst of motivation fizzles out, leaving you right where you started, only poorer in spirit and finance.

Or maybe you've even dabbled in various health supplements and holistic practices, each claiming to be the key to lasting health and vitality. But after the initial excitement wanes, you find the promises unfulfilled, as the root causes of your wellness issues remain untouched.

The truth is, you're not alone. It seems most are becoming a victim of quick fixes and fleeting trends in the health industry. These approaches are not designed to create lasting change, but rather to capitalize on your genuine desire for a better life.

That feeling of frustration, confusion, and helplessness? It's overwhelming. When you're bombarded with conflicting advice and temporary solutions, it's easy to feel lost in a sea of supposed quick fixes, none of which offer the lasting health and vitality you crave.

Here's what most don't realize: true transformation in health and energy doesn't come from a 'magic pill' or a one-size-fits-all solution. It comes from understanding the unique needs of your body and mind, and nurturing them with the right practices and habits.

And now, with the possibility of more innovative health solutions at our fingertips than ever before, it's crucial to discern the genuinely transformative approaches from the fleeting trends. This book is designed to guide you through that process.

It seems most are left in a state of perpetual anticipation, always waiting for the next big thing, yet never really achieving the health and fulfillment they yearn for. This state of limbo is not just disheartening; it's a breeding ground for deeper fears and insecurities about one's ability to lead a truly healthy life.

With "99 HACKS FOR HEALTH," we will tackle these issues head-on, empowering you to make informed, lasting changes toward a healthier, more energetic, and fulfilled life. Let's embark on this journey together.

The Cycle of Stagnation

You might be familiar with the ceaseless struggle to improve your health and vitality, to live not just longer, but better. The Cycle of Stagnation is a relentless loop that captures so many, perhaps even you, in its repetitive twists and turns. Here, we dive into each step of this draining cycle, outlining why it so often ensnares individuals striving for a healthier, more fulfilled life.

Initial Discontent Perhaps you wake up one morning and look in the mirror, not recognizing the person staring back. Maybe it's a photograph, a simple comment from a friend, or a doctor's report that triggers it. You feel a surge of motivation to change. This moment of realization is powerful, yet fraught with discomfort and dissatisfaction with your current state.

Overwhelming Options Fueled by your initial discontent, you plunge into the vast sea of health information. Detox teas, fad diets, the newest workout regimes—options are endless, and it's overwhelming. Decision fatigue sets in quickly. You try one, then another, hoping each will be the magic bullet, but nothing sticks. Confusion reigns, and your motivation begins to wane as each attempt fails to deliver lasting change.

Burst of Effort Determined, you pick a plan and throw yourself into it. For a few weeks, you are the paragon of discipline. Gym sessions, kale smoothies, meditation—perhaps you even see some early results. But the effort is immense, disproportionate to the pace of progress. It's unsustainable, and deep down, you feel this can't last.

Temporary Triumph Then, a glimpse of success. Maybe you've lost a few pounds, or you're sleeping better, feeling more energetic. It's a heady feeling, this hint of triumph. You start to believe you've finally cracked the code. Life seems brighter, and you dare to feel hopeful that maybe, just maybe, you've made it past the hurdles.

Subtle Setback But slowly, almost imperceptibly, old habits creep back in. A skipped workout here, an unhealthy meal there. The busyness of life makes it hard to maintain what you started, and the energy to keep up wanes. Before you know it, you're sliding back to where you began, disillusioned. The cycle's cruel twist is that it leaves you right where you started: staring down the same path of initial discontent.

It just goes to show that you would be wise to do something different to achieve a better, longer, healthier, more fulfilled life and stop the pain and frustration.

Which is why I'm glad you're reading this book, because as you turn the page and start reading, you will finally get the answers and insights that you're looking for.

INTRODUCTION

Imagine a life where each day brims with energy, clarity, and joy—a life where your health is not just adequate, but optimal, empowering you to live fully and freely. It's not just a distant dream; it's a tangible, achievable reality. This book is your roadmap to a healthier, more vibrant you. It doesn't matter where you are on your health journey right now; what matters is where you can go.

Part One: The Gateway to Enhanced Living

You wake up each morning, but do you wake up feeling refreshed and ready to conquer the day? Or do you drag yourself out of bed, dreading the day ahead? Your first steps in the morning can set the tone for your entire day, and indeed, your entire life. Now, imagine beginning your days with vitality, your body and mind in harmonious sync, fueled by an unseen vigor. This isn't about miraculous cures or the latest fad diets. It's about simple, profound changes that ignite profound results.

Health is the cornerstone of a fulfilling life. It's the foundation upon which everything else is built. When your health flourishes, so does your ability to enjoy life, face challenges, and pursue your dreams. Conversely, when it falters, everything you do takes more effort and yields less joy. This book is about flipping the script on your health narrative. It's about transforming your everyday habits to create a new, vibrant baseline for your life.

Part Two: The Tools for Transformation

You don't need to be a doctor, a celebrity, or an athlete to achieve exceptional health. All you need are the right tools and the resolve to use them. This guide will equip you with 99 hacks, each designed to improve how you feel and function every day. These hacks aren't just about avoiding illness; they're about creating a state of health that makes illness less likely and life more enjoyable.

Each hack has been carefully selected and tested for its effectiveness and simplicity. They don't require extraordinary resources or unsustainable sacrifices. Instead, they integrate seamlessly into the life you already lead, gently shifting your health trajectory upward. These are practical, actionable strategies that fit into your daily routine, making health improvement inevitable.

Consider how your life might change if you could systematically reduce stress, enhance your sleep quality, and nourish your body optimally. Think about the profound impact of having more mental clarity and emotional resilience. These aren't just nice-to-have qualities—they are game changers in life's complex arena. They determine how high you reach and how far you go. This book is about setting you up with everything you need to maximize your health, so you can maximize your life.

Part Three: The Road to Lifelong Vitality

Embarking on this journey might seem daunting, but remember, this isn't about a radical overnight transformation. It's about making small, consistent changes that accumulate into massive improvements over time. Like compound interest in finance, every small health investment you make pays dividends in your future well-being.

This book isn't just a read; it's a do. It's a series of stepping stones that will carry you closer to the life you want. Each chapter provides you with insights and tools that are both the motivation and the means to your ends. By applying these 90 hacks, you'll not only enhance your health; you'll enhance every aspect of your life. Energy, resilience, clarity—these are the ingredients of a life well-lived, and they're within your reach.

You might start reading this book out of curiosity. You might start with skepticism or even desperation. But regardless of where you begin, you'll finish with empowerment. You'll close the last page knowing not just more about health, but more about how to be a better version of yourself. This isn't just about what you'll achieve—it's about what you'll become.

So, take this first step with a hopeful heart and an open mind. The path to better health and a fuller life is laid out before you; all you need to do is walk it. Embrace the journey, apply the hacks, and watch as your life transforms. Welcome to a new chapter—a chapter where you live not just longer, but better.

Are you ready? Let's begin.

1

WAKE UP TO WELLNESS

"Early to bed and early to rise makes a man healthy, wealthy, and wise." - Benjamin Franklin

Morning Mastery

Kickstart your day with a series of rituals designed to boost your overall well-being right from the moment you open your eyes. 'Morning Mastery' is about setting the tone for a day filled with energy, focus, and optimum health. Let's dive into the three pillars of Morning Mastery: Hydration Rituals, Sunlight Exposure, and Mindful Breathing. By integrating these practices into your morning routine, you're not just surviving the day; you're thriving from the start.

HACK 1- Hydration Rituals

Imagine waking up after a 7-8 hour sleep. Your body has been fasting, repairing, and rebalancing. The first thing it craves isn't coffee—it's water. Starting your day with hydration can kickstart your metabolism, flush out toxins, and give your brain fuel to start functioning optimally.

Begin by drinking a large glass of water (around 500 ml) as soon as you wake up. If you want to take it up a notch, consider lukewarm water with a squeeze of fresh lemon. This isn't just about quenching thirst; it's a ritual to reactivate your digestive system gently and naturally. Lemon water is also a good source of vitamin C, perfect for boosting your immune system.

For those looking to enhance this ritual further, a pinch of Himalayan salt or a teaspoon of apple cider vinegar can be added to the mix. Both are touted for their health benefits, including aiding digestion and balancing blood sugar levels.

HACK 2- Sunlight Exposure

Once you've hydrated, it's time to seek out sunlight. Exposing yourself to natural light first thing in the morning can have profound effects on your body. It helps to regulate your body's internal clock, or circadian rhythm, which not only improves your sleep quality but also enhances your mood and energy levels throughout the day.

Try to get at least 10-15 minutes of morning sun. If you're an early riser, this is a serene time to embrace the calmness of the morning while filling your sensory inputs with natural light. This exposure helps halt the production of melatonin (the sleep hormone) and kickstarts the production of serotonin (the happy hormone), setting a positive mood tone for the day.

For those living in less sunny locales or finding themselves in the darker months, consider a light therapy lamp. These devices can mimic natural sunlight and are an effective tool for maintaining a steady circadian rhythm.

HACK 3- Mindful Breathing

With your body hydrated and basking in sunlight, it's now perfect timing to engage in mindful breathing. This practice is about more than just taking deep breaths; it's about becoming acutely aware of your breathing pattern and using it to centre your mind for the day ahead.

Start with a simple technique: the 4-7-8 method. Breathe in through your nose for 4 seconds, hold that breath for 7 seconds, and exhale slowly through your mouth for 8 seconds. This method not only reduces anxiety but also helps lower blood pressure and provides a sense of calm.

Incorporating mindful breathing into your morning can enhance mental clarity and emotional resilience. Practicing it daily strengthens your mindfulness muscle, making you more present and engaged throughout the day. It's a tool that empowers you to handle stress more effectively and maintain peace in both your mind and body.

As you integrate these elements into your morning, you'll notice a shift not only in your physical health but also in your mental and emotional well-being. 'Morning Mastery' isn't just about jumping out of bed and rushing through a routine; it's about setting a deliberate tone that promotes sustained energy, focus, and presence. It's about starting your day with intentional practices that nourish and prepare you for the challenges and joys that lie ahead.

Remember, the key to benefiting from Morning Mastery is consistency. Make these practices a non-negotiable part of your morning, and watch as your days transform – becoming more productive, joyful, and healthy. Each morning is a new opportunity to enhance your well-being, so embrace these rituals and reclaim your life, one sunrise at a time.

Power Breakfasts

HACK 4- Protein-Packed Start

If you've ever wondered whether what you gulp down for breakfast can really set the tone for your day, the answer is a resounding "yes." Let's dive into the world of protein-rich breakfasts and uncover why upping your morning protein can be a game-changer for your health and energy levels.

Protein, an essential macronutrient, is often dubbed the building block of life. Consuming protein in the morning can help stabilize your blood sugar levels, reduce cravings for sugary snacks, and prevent overeating later in the day. It's not just about the quantity but the quality of the protein that counts.

Start with eggs – versatile, affordable, and packed with high-quality protein. Scrambled, poached, or boiled, eggs can be a canvas for a variety of flavors and ingredients. Throw in some spinach for iron and mushrooms for vitamin D, or if you're feeling adventurous, a sprinkle of turmeric or chili flakes can add a new dimension of flavor and health benefits.

For those who lean towards plant-based diets, fear not. Options like chia seeds, hemp seeds, and quinoa are not only high in protein but also provide essential amino acids that your body can't produce on its own. A simple chia pudding, made by soaking the seeds in almond milk overnight and topping with berries and a drizzle of honey, can be a delightful and nutritious start to your day.

Lastly, don't forget Greek yoghurt. It's a powerhouse of protein, packed with probiotics that aid digestion and enhance gut health. Mix it with a handful of nuts for healthy fats and sprinkle some antioxidant-rich blueberries on top for a balanced, protein-packed breakfast that will keep you energized and satisfied.

HACK 5- Smoothie Science

The art of blending a smoothie is like conducting a symphony; the ingredients need to harmonize to create a balance of flavor and nutrition. Smoothies are not only quick and easy to make but also a brilliant way to get a concentrated dose of nutrients first thing in the morning.

Start with the base. While water or ice can do, consider unsweetened almond milk, coconut water, or kefir for added flavor and health benefits. Almond milk provides a creamy texture without the heaviness of dairy, coconut water offers hydration and potassium, and kefir brings in probiotics for a gut health boost.

Next, pick your protein. A scoop of whey or a plant-based protein powder can ensure you're getting your morning protein fix. If you prefer whole foods, silken tofu, Greek yoghurt, or a spoonful of nut butter can be excellent protein sources.

Now, for the fruits and vegetables – the real MVPs of your smoothie. Spinach, kale, and avocado blend nicely and offer loads of nutrients without overpowering the taste. Combine them with high-antioxidant fruits like berries, mango, or banana for natural sweetness and a fiber boost.

Don't forget to add some superfoods for an extra nutrient kick. A teaspoon of spirulina adds a burst of vitamins and minerals, while flaxseeds or hemp seeds sprinkle in omega-3 fatty acids essential for brain health.

Finally, tailor your smoothie to your taste and health needs. Need a boost in immunity? Add a dash of turmeric or ginger. Looking for extra energy? A spoonful of maca powder can do the trick. The beauty of smoothies lies in their versatility, so feel free to experiment with different combinations to find what works best for you.

HACK 6- Oats for Energy

Oats are the unsung hero of the breakfast table. Not only are they packed with fiber, which can help maintain a healthy digestive system, but they also offer a fantastic energy boost that's slow-releasing, keeping you full and focused throughout the morning.

The simplest way to enjoy oats is in the form of porridge. Cooking oats slowly and topping them with fruits and seeds can transform them into a comforting yet nutritious meal. To maximize the health benefits, opt for steel-cut or rolled oats, as they undergo less processing than their instant counterparts.

For a richer taste and added protein, cook your oats in milk or a milk alternative instead of water. This not only enhances the flavor but also contributes to the creaminess of the porridge. Sweeten naturally with ripe bananas, a splash of maple syrup, or a handful of dried fruits.

If you're always on the go, overnight oats can be a lifesaver. Simply mix rolled oats with milk or Greek yoghurt, add some chia seeds for extra fiber, and let them soak in the fridge overnight. In the morning, top with fresh fruits, nuts, or a dollop of nut butter for a quick, transportable, and hearty breakfast.

For those who like a bit of crunch, homemade granola can be a great alternative. Combine oats with a mix of nuts, seeds, and a little honey or agave nectar, then bake until golden. The result? A delicious and crunchy topping that's perfect over yoghurt or mixed into a smoothie bowl.

Whether you choose porridge, overnight oats, or granola, incorporating oats into your morning routine is a surefire way to boost your energy levels and start your day off right.

Early Bird Exercise

HACK 7- Stretching Basics

Imagine this: the birds are just starting to chirp, the world outside is bathed in a soft, early morning light, and you, my friend, are gently preparing your body to face the day ahead. Stretching first thing in the morning sounds simple, but its benefits are anything but minimal. It's like sending a love letter to your muscles and joints, thanking them in advance for the day's work.

Starting with some basic stretches does more than just wake

up your muscles; it increases your blood flow, improves your posture, and boosts your energy levels. Here's how to get into the groove:

Begin with a full-body stretch. Lie on your back, reach your arms overhead and stretch your legs out. Imagine someone is gently pulling your hands and feet in opposite directions. Hold this for about 15 to 30 seconds. This is not just any stretch; it's a signal to your body that the day has begun.

Next, target your neck and shoulders. Tilt your head towards your shoulder, using your hand to gently pull. After about 15 seconds, switch sides. Why bother? Because these are areas where stress likes to throw a party. By doing these stretches, you're shutting down that party before it even starts.

Don't forget your lower body. Stand up and gently pull one foot towards your buttock, keeping your knees together and pushing your hip forward. This stretches your quadriceps, a key muscle group for anyone who plans on walking more than just from the bed to the breakfast table.

Incorporate these stretches into a 5-minute routine, and you'll not only limber up but also kick-start your metabolism. It's like warming up your car on a chilly morning – everything runs a bit smoother afterwards.

HACK 8- Short HIIT Session

High-Intensity Interval Training (HIIT) might sound intimidating, but it's actually perfect for any fitness level. The beauty of HIIT is its adaptability and efficiency. In just a few minutes, you can achieve what might take 30 minutes of moderate-paced exercise. It's about working smarter, not longer.

A basic HIIT session in the morning can set a tone of achievement for your day. You're stacking up victories while others are still snoozing their alarms. Here's a simple 10-minute routine you can do at home, no equipment needed:

Start with 30 seconds of jumping jacks. This isn't just a throwback to your school days; it's an explosive movement that wakes up every part of the body

Follow up with 20 seconds of rest. Breathe

Move on to 30 seconds of squats. Keep your back straight and chest up. This engages your core and lower body

Another 20 seconds rest. Catch your breath

Do 30 seconds of high knees. Pump your arms and lift those knees. This increases your heart rate and improves overall agility

Rest for 20 seconds

Finish with 30 seconds of push-ups. Modify them by dropping to your knees if needed. This strengthens your upper body and core.

Repeat this circuit twice. By the end, you will have boosted your metabolism, improved your endurance, and sharpened your mental focus. All within the time it might take to scroll through your morning social media feed.

HACK 9- Morning Walk Benefits

Rounding off your morning exercise with a walk might seem too simple to be effective, but never underestimate the power of a good walk. Walking in the morning is like a tonic for the mind and body. It's a gentle yet powerful way to increase your fitness, clear your mind, and prepare yourself for the day ahead.

A brisk 20-minute walk after your stretches or HIIT session can help to cool down your body and set your mind at ease. Walking isn't just about moving from point A to B; it's a meditative practice that connects you with your environment and your own thoughts.

During your walk, pay attention to your surroundings, the rhythm of your steps, the feeling of the air on your skin, and the sounds around you. This mindfulness element reduces stress levels and anxiety, setting a calm, composed tone for your day.

Moreover, exposure to natural light in the morning helps to

regulate your body's internal clock, enhancing sleep quality at night. Better sleep leads to better mornings, creating a virtuous cycle of wellness.

Incorporating walking into your morning routine also has long-term benefits, including improved cardiovascular health and better weight management. It's a low-impact exercise that keeps you physically active without the wear and tear that other, more intense workouts might impose.

In short, by starting your day with some basic stretches, a short burst of HIIT, and a rejuvenating walk, you're not just priming yourself for today; you're investing in a healthier, more energetic future. It's about setting the tone for a life where you're not just surviving each day but thriving. So lace up those trainers, and let's make each morning a stepping stone to a better life.

RECAP AND ACTION ITEMS FOR THE 9 WAKE UP TO WELLNESS HACKS

Congratulations on completing your journey through the "Wake Up to Wellness" segment of our book. By now, you've equipped yourself with the knowledge to kick-start your mornings in a way that sets the tone for a healthier, more vibrant day. Let's quickly recap the essentials and lay out some concrete steps you can take to integrate these insights into your daily routine.

Starting your day with the Morning Mastery techniques, you've learned the importance of rehydrating your body after a night's sleep, soaking up some morning sunlight to reset your internal clock, and using mindful breathing to reduce stress and center your thoughts. Each of these practices plays a crucial role in optimizing your body and mind for the day ahead.

Next, in Power Breakfasts, we explored how a protein-packed start can support muscle health and keep you feeling fuller longer, the benefits of crafting nutrient-rich smoothies, and how incorporating oats can provide you with sustained energy. These food choices not only nourish your body but also sharpen your mental clarity and focus.

Lastly, the Early Bird Exercise section underscored the value of gentle stretching to awaken your muscles, a short HIIT session to boost your metabolism, and the myriad benefits of a morning walk, including enhancing mood and improving cardiovascular health.

Action Items:

Hydrate First Thing:

Tomorrow morning, start your day with a large glass of water—perhaps with a slice of lemon for an extra vitamin C boost

Sunlight and Breathing:

Set a reminder to spend a few minutes outside in natural sunlight and perform a brief mindful breathing exercise. Even just five minutes can have a profound impact

Protein-Packed Breakfast:

Plan your meals tonight so tomorrow's breakfast includes a good source of protein—think eggs, Greek yoghurt, or a scoop of protein powder in your smoothie

Experiment with Oats and Smoothies:

This week, try different types of oats and smoothie recipes to find your favorites. Keep it interesting by varying the fruits, nuts, and seeds you add

Incorporate Morning Exercise:

Alternate between stretching, a quick HIIT workout, and a brisk walk in the mornings. Start with at least one of these activities daily and build up as you establish your routine.

By consistently applying these strategies every morning, you'll not only feel more energized and focused but also set a positive tone that can lead to making healthier choices throughout the day. Remember, the goal is to make incremental changes that together result in a significant impact on your well-being. Here's to living a healthier, longer, and more fulfilled life!

2

MENTAL CLARITY THROUGH MINIMALISM

"Out of clutter, find simplicity. From discord, find harmony. In the middle of difficulty lies opportunity." - Albert Einstein

Declutter Your Space

In the quest for mental clarity and a profoundly fulfilling life, the physical spaces around us play an underrated role. The environment you inhabit can either boost your mental energy or drain it. To harness the full potential of minimalism, let's start where you spend most of your waking hours: your space.

HACK 10- Benefits of a Minimal Workspace

Imagine entering a workspace that's both visually and functionally serene. Surfaces are clear, each item has a purpose, and there's an inherent sense of order. This isn't just an aesthete's dream—it's a recipe for enhanced mental clarity.

A minimal workspace reduces cognitive overload. With fewer distractions, your brain isn't jumping from one stimulus to another. Research suggests that visual clutter competes for your attention, leading to decreased performance and increased stress. Conversely, a minimalist environment promotes a sharper focus and a faster retrieval of information. This means you can concentrate better, process information quicker, and ultimately, perform at your peak.

Moreover, a decluttered workspace can lead to heightened creativity. With the unnecessary stripped away, there's more mental space to think broadly and generate innovative ideas. It's about making room for creativity to flourish by removing the physical and mental clutter that stifles it.

HACK 11- Daily Decluttering Techniques

Decluttering isn't a one-off task; it's a continuous process. To maintain a minimal workspace, integrate decluttering into your daily routine. Here are some effective techniques:

Start with a clean slate:

Each day, begin with a clear desk. Last day's remnants—be it papers, cups, or tech gadgets—should be cleared away. This sets a calm tone for the day and signals your brain that it's time to focus.

Adopt the one-minute rule:

If a task can be done in a minute or less, do it immediately. This could be anything from filing a document to replying to an email. Keeping on top of these small tasks prevents them from piling up and cluttering your physical and mental space.

Use minimal stationary:

Limit the number of pens, notebooks, and other desk items to what's essential. Each item on your desk should earn its place by being functional or providing real value to your work.

Digitize where possible:

Reduce paper clutter by digitizing documents. Not only does this clear physical space, but it also makes information retrieval quicker and easier, thereby enhancing productivity.

End your day with a 10-minute tidy:

Spend the last few minutes of your workday resetting your space. This not only prepares your desk for the next day but also gives you a small sense of closure, signaling to your brain that the working day is done.

HACK 12- Digital Detox Tips

In today's hyper-connected world, digital clutter can be just as overwhelming as physical clutter. Emails, notifications, and endless apps can scatter your focus and dilute your productivity. Here are some tips to help you detox digitally:

Implement an email schedule:

Rather than checking emails continuously throughout the day, set specific times for this task. This could be mid-morning, after lunch, and late afternoon. Outside these times, keep your email closed to avoid distractions.

Turn off non-essential notifications:

Every ping or buzz pulls your attention away from the task at hand. Dive into your settings and disable notifications for anything that isn't essential to your work or well-being.

Use technology mindfully:

Be intentional about your technology use. Ask yourself whether each device or app serves a purpose that aligns with your goals and values. If not, it might be time to let it go.

Embrace 'single-tasking':

When working on a device, try to keep only one window or app open at a time. This promotes deeper focus and reduces the urge to multi-task, which can be mentally exhausting.

Regular digital clean-ups:

Set a monthly reminder to go through your digital files and apps. Unsubscribe from newsletters you no longer read, delete apps you don't use, and clear out redundant files. This not only frees up space on your devices but also declutters your mind.

By adopting these practices, you can create a workspace that not only boosts your productivity but also enhances your overall well-being. Remember, the goal of minimalism isn't just to have less for the sake of less. It's about making more room for what truly matters—your health, your peace of mind, and your journey towards a fulfilling life.

Simplify Your Diet

HACK 13- Eating Whole Foods

Let's kick off with a profound, yet beautifully simple strategy: eating whole foods. Imagine your diet as a clean, uncluttered workspace where everything you need is within easy reach, nothing unnecessary in sight. That's what whole foods can do for your body and mind.

Whole foods are items that remain close to their natural state: think fresh fruits, vegetables, nuts, seeds, whole grains, and lean meats. They are free from additives, colorings, and preservatives that can cloud your mental clarity. By incorporating more whole foods into your diet, you are not only fueling your body with the best nutrients but also simplifying the process of choosing what to eat.

When shopping, aim to spend most of your time around the perimeter of the grocery store. This is typically where the freshest foods are kept. The middle aisles generally contain the processed foods, which you want to avoid. Try to pick items with the shortest ingredient lists — if it reads like a chemistry experiment, it's probably not the best choice for maintaining clear mental function.

HACK 14- Meal Planning

Now, onto meal planning — a true minimalist tactic to reduce daily decisions and increase efficiency. By planning your meals, you avoid the mental fatigue of making multiple food-related decisions throughout the day, which can lead to better diet choices and a clearer mind.

Start simple: plan just one meal a day and gradually increase as you become more comfortable with the process. Perhaps begin with dinner, as it can often be the most complex meal to prepare. Write down a weekly menu and shop accordingly. This not only helps you avoid buying unnecessary items but ensures you have all the ingredients you need, reducing last-minute trips to the store.

A good tip is to prepare portions in advance. Cooking a batch of quinoa or roasting a tray of vegetables on a Sunday can save you considerable time during the week. These can easily be turned into different meals by adding varying proteins or dressings, keeping your diet interesting and varied.

HACK 15- Avoiding Processed Foods

Finally, a critical aspect of simplifying your diet is avoiding processed foods. These are often packed with hidden sugars, unhealthy fats, and a barrage of chemicals that can do more harm than good. Not only can these foods impact your physical health, but they also have the potential to cloud your mental clarity.

Start by reading labels meticulously. If sugar, or any of its numerous aliases (think high fructose corn syrup, agave nectar, etc.), appears in the first few ingredients, it's best to steer clear. Also, be wary of anything that claims to be an 'instant' version of a traditionally slow-cooked dish — these products are typically loaded with preservatives and artificial flavorings.

Instead, focus on food items that contribute to sustained energy levels and support brain function. Foods rich in omega-3 fatty acids, such as salmon and flaxseeds, are excellent for this. Similarly, antioxidants found in berries and leafy greens help combat oxidative stress, promoting clearer thinking.

By simplifying your diet and focusing on these key elements — eating whole foods, planning your meals, and avoiding processed items — you set yourself up for a clearer, more focused mental state. It's about making mindful choices that nourish both your body and mind, paving the way for a healthier, more fulfilled life. Embrace the minimalist approach in your eating habits and watch how it positively affects your overall clarity and wellbeing.

Streamline Your Thoughts

HACK 16- Journaling for Clarity

Let's kick off with something you've probably heard about a thousand times but might not have truly given a shot: journaling. Now, before you roll your eyes and skip ahead, hear this out. Journaling isn't just about documenting your day or your travels; it's a potent tool for mental decluttering and gaining clarity in the chaos of everyday life.

Imagine dumping all the buzzing thoughts from your brain onto a page. Sounds relieving, right? That's what journaling can do. It helps you clear out mental clutter, making room for more structured and creative thinking. Start with the basics: grab a notebook and write down whatever comes to mind. Don't worry about coherence or style—this isn't for anyone's eyes but yours.

To refine your journaling into a clarity tool, consider these strategies:-

Morning Pages: Right after you wake up, write three pages of whatever pops into your head. This practice, popularized by Julia Cameron, isn't about crafting beautiful prose; it's about clearing your mind for the day ahead

Gratitude Journaling: Each night, jot down three things you were grateful for that day. This not only steers your focus towards positive elements in your life but also reduces stress and boosts your mood

Problem-solving Entries: Whenever you're faced with a dilemma, use your journal to work through possible solutions. Writing down pros and cons or various scenarios can help you see answers that aren't always apparent when you're just pondering them in your head.

The key here is consistency. The more regularly you journal, the more natural it will become and the clearer your thoughts will be. It's like any form of exercise; the benefits accumulate and become more apparent over time.

HACK 17- Meditation Practices

Next up, let's demystify meditation. Often wrapped in an aura of mystique, the core of meditation is quite simple: it's about being present. In our hyper-connected world, where our attention is a currency in constant demand, giving yourself the gift of presence is revolutionary.

Meditation starts with focusing on your breath or a mantra — a word or phrase repeated to aid concentration. But if sitting silently sounds too daunting, there are numerous other forms you can explore:-

Guided Meditations:

These are perfect if you're just starting out. You can find countless guided sessions online that can help steer your focus away from the whirlwind of daily thoughts

Mindfulness Meditation:

This involves being intensely aware of what you're sensing and feeling at every moment, without interpretation or judgment. It teaches you to observe your thoughts passing by like cars on a street, without getting hitched to any particular one

Walking Meditation:

If sitting still isn't your thing, try meditating while walking. Focus on the sensation of your feet touching the ground, the rhythm of your breath, and the sounds around you. It's meditative multitasking at its best.

Remember, the goal of meditation isn't to empty your mind but rather to become aware of your thoughts without getting entangled in them. It's about finding a bit of stillness in the storm, which, believe it or not, can dramatically enhance your clarity and focus.

HACK 18- Setting Intentions

Finally, let's talk about setting intentions. While goals are generally outcome-focused, intentions are more about the journey — the values and energies you want to bring into your daily activities. Setting intentions is like creating a mental blueprint for how you want to engage with the world around you.

Each morning, take a few minutes to reflect on what qualities you want to cultivate for the day. Maybe it's patience during a meeting, creativity for a project, or just being more present with your loved ones. Here's how to make intention-setting impactful:

Be Specific:

Vague intentions are less likely to stick. Be as specific as possible. Instead of "be more present," try "actively listen without interrupting in conversations today."

Write It Down:

There's power in penning it down. Write your daily intentions in your journal. It serves as a reminder throughout the day and reinforces your commitment

Reflect:

At the end of the day, spend a few minutes reflecting on how well you aligned with your intentions. This isn't about judging yourself but rather observing and learning from your experiences.

Setting intentions helps to direct your mental energy where it's most valuable, reducing wasteful scatter and aligning your actions with your values. It's a minimalistic approach to managing your mental space, ensuring that you're focusing on what truly matters to you.

By integrating these practices into your life — journaling for clarity, meditating for presence, and setting intentions for purposeful living — you're not just clearing out mental clutter; you're actively designing a mindset that embraces simplicity and clarity. Streamlining your thoughts isn't just about reducing the noise; it's about amplifying what truly enriches your life.

RECAP AND ACTION ITEMS ON THE 9 MENTAL CLARITY THROUGH MINIMALISM HACKS

By now, you've travelled through a transformative journey of decluttering your space, simplifying your diet, and streamlining your thoughts. Each step is designed to lead you towards a clearer, more focused mindset, empowering you to live a healthier, more fulfilled life.

Declutter Your Space

The environment you inhabit directly influences your mental clarity. A minimal workspace isn't just aesthetically pleasing; it reduces stress and boosts productivity. Begin by removing unnecessary items from your work area. Commit to a daily routine of tidying up before you finish your day so that each morning welcomes you with a clean slate. Additionally, take proactive steps to detox from digital clutter. Limit social media usage and unsubscribe from unnecessary emails to reduce digital noise.

Simplify Your Diet

What you eat has a profound effect on how you feel and function. Embrace whole foods and plan your meals to include a variety of fruits, vegetables, whole grains, and lean proteins. This approach not only nourishes your body but also your mind by stabilizing blood sugar and enhancing mood. Steer clear of processed foods as much as possible to avoid the mental fog and lethargy associated with high sugar and high-fat diets.

Streamline Your Thoughts

Your thoughts shape your reality. Begin each day by journaling; it's a powerful tool to clarify your thoughts and emotions, setting a positive tone for the day. Incorporate meditation into your daily routine to cultivate a state of mindfulness, which helps in managing stress and enhancing focus. Finally, set clear intentions for what you want to achieve each day, week, or month. This practice keeps you aligned with your goals and ensures that your actions are purposeful.

Action Steps:

- Start each morning by clearing your workspace and planning a whole-food-based meal

- Spend at least 10 minutes journaling to organize your thoughts and another 10 minutes in meditation to center your mind

- At the end of each day, review your intentions to assess your progress and prepare for the next day.

Remember, minimalism is not about having less for the sake of less; it's about making room for more of what matters. By adopting these practices, you're not just decluttering your space or diet, but you're decluttering your life, paving the way for enhanced health, energy, and mental clarity. Embrace the journey, and watch how these small changes add up to significant transformations.

3

BEAT STRESS BEFORE IT BEGINS

"It's not stress that kills us, it is our reaction to it." – *Hans Selye*

Recognize Stress Signals

Stress: it's like that uninvited guest at your party who not only crashes but also refuses to leave. Recognizing the early signals of stress is crucial because, let's face it, once stress settles in, it can throw your whole system out of whack. Understanding what triggers your stress, along with recognizing its physical and emotional indicators, is the first step towards managing it effectively. So, let's dive in and unpack these signals, helping you to stay two steps ahead of stress.

HACK 19- Understanding Your Stress Triggers

Imagine you're a detective in your own psychological thriller, where the mystery to solve is what triggers your stress. Triggers are unique as fingerprints; what might send you into a spiral may not even bother someone else. Common triggers include work deadlines, financial worries, or personal conflicts, but the subtler ones often go unnoticed until they pack a punch.

Start by keeping a stress diary. Every time you feel stressed, jot down the event that preceded it. Was it a comment from a colleague, a certain part of your day, or maybe even something as simple as skipping a meal? Over time, patterns emerge. You might notice that your stress spikes during your weekly meeting with your boss or when you're handling too many tasks at once.

Understanding your triggers is like mapping the minefield of your daily life; once you know where the mines are, you can navigate more safely. Awareness is your first tool in preemptively managing stress. By recognizing what sets you off, you can start to put measures in place to either avoid these triggers or dampen their impact on your life.

HACK 20- Physical Signs of Stress

Your body often knows you're stressed before your mind catches up. Physical signs of stress are the body's alarm bells, and they can be as loud as a siren if you're attuned to them. Common physical indicators include headaches, muscle tension or pain, chest pain, fatigue, and changes in sex drive. More subtle signs might include stomach upset, sleep disturbances or a change in appetite.

Listen to your body; it's smarter than you might give it credit for. For instance, if you find your jaw clenched and your shoulders up around your ears while checking emails, that's a physical manifestation of stress. Or maybe you notice that you always get a headache after a prolonged period of financial planning.

Once you start noticing these signs, you can take quick action to alleviate them before they lead to more severe stress responses. Simple things like changing your posture, taking a few deep breaths, or even stepping away from your desk for a few minutes can help reset your physical state and prevent stress from escalating.

HACK 21 - Emotional Indicators

While physical signs of stress are easier to identify, emotional signs can be a bit trickier. They often manifest as irritability, feeling overwhelmed, mood swings, or a general sense of anxiety. You might find yourself less patient than usual, quick to frustration or suddenly feeling teary for little or no apparent reason.

These emotional indicators are telling you that your mental bandwidth is being stretched too thin. It's important to address these feelings head-on rather than brushing them aside. Acknowledging your emotional state gives you a chance to adjust your course and implement strategies to lighten your emotional load.

For example, feeling overwhelmed might be a cue to review and prioritize your commitments. Maybe it's time to delegate, or perhaps say no to additional responsibilities. Addressing your emotional state isn't just about coping with stress; it's about creating a more sustainable lifestyle that allows for emotional fluctuations without letting them capsize your boat.

Recognizing stress signals is all about tuning into your body and mind and listening to the subtle cues they provide. Like a seasoned sailor who reads the wind and waves, understanding your stress triggers and signs—both physical and emotional—enables you to navigate through turbulent waters with greater ease and resilience. By becoming more aware of these signals, you empower yourself to manage stress proactively, keeping its impacts at bay and maintaining your overall health and wellbeing.

Quick Stress Relief Techniques

When stress knocks on your door with its not-so-gentle ways, wouldn't it be great to have a toolkit ready to combat it swiftly? Here, we delve into simple yet effective techniques that can help dissipate stress quickly, ensuring it doesn't spiral out of control.

HACK 22- Breathing Exercises

One of the most immediate ways to tackle stress is to change the way you breathe. It sounds almost too simple, doesn't it? But under stress, our breathing pattern changes. Typically, the breath becomes shallow and quick. Reversing this consciously can drastically reduce stress.

Let's start with a technique you can do anywhere – the 4-6-8 breathing method. Begin by exhaling completely through your mouth. Close your lips, and inhale silently through your nose as you count to four. Hold your breath for a count of six. Then, exhale completely through your mouth, making a whoosh sound to a count of eight. This one complete breath will help calm the nervous system. Repeat this cycle at least four times.

Why does this work? When you breathe deeply, it sends a message to your brain to calm down and relax. The brain then sends this message to your body. Such breathing exercises can have immediate effects in relieving stress, not only mentally but also physically.

Next, explore the abdominal breathing technique. Place one hand on your chest and the other on your belly. Take a deep breath in through the nose, ensuring the diaphragm inflates with enough air to create a stretch in the lungs. Aim for six to ten deep, slow breaths per minute for ten minutes each day to experience immediate reductions to heart rate and blood pressure. Keep this practice up, and you might find the benefits extend much beyond immediate stress relief.

HACK 23- Progressive Muscle Relaxation

Another fantastic method to release stress on the spot is Progressive Muscle Relaxation (PMR). This technique involves tensing each muscle group but doing so very deliberately and then relaxing them equally deliberately. It's like pressing a reset button on your body's stress levels.

Start by finding a comfortable place where you can either sit or lie down. Take a few deep breaths before you begin. Then, focus on tensing the muscles in your toes for about five seconds and then relax them for 30 seconds. Progressively work your way up through your body—the legs, abdomen, chest, arms, and neck. Not only does this help relieve tension, but it also helps you become more aware of your physical sensations, which can be particularly useful when your body is responding to stress.

The beauty of PMR is that it can be done in many settings, whether you're at home or in a quiet corner of your workplace. Over time, this method can help reduce overall tension and stress, improve sleep, and enhance your overall sense of well-being.

HACK 24- Listening to Music

Now, let's turn the dial up on your mood with some music. Listening to music has a remarkably relaxing effect on the mind and body, especially slow, quiet classical music. This type of music can have a beneficial effect on your physiological functions, slowing the pulse and heart rate, lowering blood pressure, and decreasing the levels of stress hormones.

However, classical music isn't everyone's cup of tea. The key is to listen to music that you love. The sounds of ocean waves, the rustle of leaves in a forest, or even a track from your favorite artist can reduce cortisol levels, which is a common stress marker.

Create a playlist of songs or sounds that evoke happiness or calm within you. Turn to this playlist whenever you feel stress creeping up. Let the music carry you away from your immediate worries and help anchor you in the present moment.

By integrating these quick stress relief techniques into your life, you can begin to handle stress more effectively as it arises. Each method serves as a powerful tool to not just manage stress, but to enhance your overall quality of life. Remember, the goal is not to eliminate stress entirely—such a pursuit would be futile—but to manage it in such a way that it doesn't manage you.

Long-Term Stress Management

HACK 25- Regular Exercise

Imagine incorporating a habit into your life that not only chisels your body but also sharpens your mind, boosting your mood while barricading it against stress. That's what regular exercise does. When you engage in physical activity, your body releases endorphins—those are the chemicals in your brain that act as natural painkillers and mood elevators. They're often referred to as the 'feel-good' hormones.

The beauty of exercise is its versatility in form and function. Whether it's a brisk walk in the park, a sweaty home workout session, or a calming yoga routine, the key is consistency. Aim for at least150 minutes of moderate aerobic activity or 75 minutes of vigorous activity each week, as recommended by health experts. But more importantly, choose activities that you enjoy. If you love what you do, it's easier to stick to it, and the benefits on your stress levels are more pronounced.

Regular exercise also helps you with better sleep, which is often disrupted by stress. When your body is physically tired, your sleep quality improves, turning into a natural stress reducer. Additionally, engaging in group sports can provide a social aspect that further aids stress relief, connecting you with others and fostering a sense of community.

HACK 26- Healthy Social Interactions

Speaking of community, never underestimate the power of healthy social interactions in managing stress. Humans are inherently social creatures, and isolation can exacerbate stress. Engaging with friends, family, or even pets provides valuable emotional support, helping to distract you from daily pressures and anchoring your reality towards positive stimuli.

However, it's crucial to choose your company wisely. Surround yourself with positive and supportive people. They create an environment where you can speak openly about your feelings and frustrations, which is a critical outlet for relieving stress. On the flip side, toxic relationships do the exact opposite, often increasing the stress you are trying to manage.

If face-to-face interactions are challenging, technology offers a plethora of options. Video calls, social media, and even old-fashioned phone calls can help bridge the gap. Also, consider joining clubs or groups that align with your interests. Whether it's a book club, a hiking group, or a volunteer organization, these social structures support engagement and provide a sense of belonging and purpose, all of which are excellent for stress control.

HACK 27- Time Management Skills

Finally, let's talk about time management—a critical area often overlooked in stress management. The feeling of being overwhelmed is frequently a symptom of poor time management. By enhancing your skills in this area, you can transform your day from a chaos-ridden sprint to a well-paced marathon with enough time for everything, including breaks.

Start by prioritizing tasks. Not every item on your to-do list needs immediate attention. Learn to differentiate between what is urgent and what is important. Tools like the Eisenhower Box can be incredibly helpful in this regard, helping you decide on and prioritize tasks by urgency and importance.

Once your tasks are prioritized, create a structured schedule. Allocate specific times for each task, including time for breaks. The Pomodoro Technique, where you work for 25 minutes and then take a 5-minute break, can significantly enhance your productivity and manage stress. During your breaks, resist the urge to scroll through social media or check emails. Instead, do something truly relaxing like stretching, a quick walk, or just closing your eyes and breathing deeply.

Effective time management also means learning to say no. You don't have to accept every request that comes your way. Assess your priorities and make decisions based on what aligns best with your goals and personal well-being.

By integrating these strategies into your life—regular physical activity that you enjoy, nurturing positive social interactions, and mastering time management—you equip yourself with a robust set of tools for managing stress long-term. Each element not only helps reduce stress but also enhances your overall quality of life, contributing to a healthier, happier you. Consider these strategies as part of an ongoing commitment to your well-being. Just like any other skill, they require practice and dedication, but the payoff—a vibrant, energetic, and fulfilled life—is well worth the effort.

RECAP AND ACTION ITEMS ON THE 9 BEAT STRESS BEFORE IT BEGINS HACKS

Congratulations on completing this vital chapter on managing and overcoming stress. By now, you've gained the tools to recognize stress signals, engage in quick relief techniques, and implement long-term strategies to manage stress effectively.

Stress is inevitable, but how you handle it can transform your health and energy levels, ultimately enhancing your life quality. Let's put these insights into practice with some actionable steps.

Journal Your Stress Triggers:

Start by keeping a stress diary. Over the next week, jot down moments when you feel stressed, noting what triggered the stress and how you reacted. This will help you understand your personal stress patterns and prepare you to handle them better.

Practice Breathing Exercises:

Each morning, or when you feel stress creeping in, take a minute to perform a simple breathing exercise: Inhale deeply for a count of four, hold for a count of four, and exhale for a count of four. This practice can center your mind and reduce immediate stress.

Incorporate Progressive Muscle Relaxation:

Commit to a 10-minute session of progressive muscle relaxation before bed. Systematically tense and then relax different muscle groups. This not only helps in reducing physical tension but also aids in better sleep.

Create a Playlist:

Music can be a powerful ally against stress. Create a playlist of tracks that lift your spirits or calm your mind. Turn to this playlist whenever you need a quick emotional boost.

Schedule Regular Exercise:

Aim for at least 150 minutes of moderate aerobic activity or 75 minutes of vigorous activity each week, as recommended by health experts. Exercise is a proven stress buster and mood lifter.

Foster Healthy Relationships:

Make it a point to connect with friends and family regularly. Social support is crucial for managing stress and maintaining psychological well-being.

Improve Your Time Management:

Assess how you spend your time daily. Identify periods where you can cut down on unnecessary activities to reduce rush and create buffers for relaxation.

By integrating these strategies into your daily life, you're not just combating stress; you're setting the stage for a healthier, more energetic, and fulfilling life. Remember, the goal is not to eliminate stress entirely but to manage it so effectively that it no longer controls your life. Take it one step at a time, and soon, you'll find yourself mastering the art of stress management.

4

OPTIMISE YOUR SLEEP

"Sleep is the best meditation." – *Dalai Lama*

Creating a Sleep Sanctuary

Transforming your bedroom into a sleep sanctuary is one of the most impactful steps you can take towards improving your nightly rest. Think of it as crafting a retreat that naturally invites relaxation and rest, a personal haven that speaks the language of sleep. Here, we'll delve into how you can optimize your bedroom environment, choose the right mattress, and manage blue light exposure to significantly enhance your sleep quality.

HACK 28- Ideal Bedroom Environment

The environment you sleep in profoundly influences your ability to drift off effortlessly and stay asleep throughout the night. Your bedroom should be a sensory-relief zone, optimized for calm and comfort. Start with the basics: temperature, noise, and light.

Temperature:

Keeping your bedroom at a cool temperature, ideally between 16-18°C, can significantly enhance the quality of your sleep. A cooler room helps decrease your body's core temperature, signaling to your body that it's time to sleep. Consider investing in a thermostat that can maintain this optimal temperature throughout the night or even a fan for a gentle breeze.

Noise:

Noise can be a major disruptor of sleep. If you live in a noisy neighborhood or share your home, consider using a white noise machine to mask disruptive sounds. Earplugs can also be an effective solution. The key is consistency in the soundscape of your bedroom; sudden noises are more likely to wake you than a consistent hum.

Light:

Light exposure plays a crucial role in regulating your sleep-wake cycle. Blackout curtains or heavy blinds can block external light sources, such as streetlights or an early sunrise, which might otherwise interfere with your sleep. This simple change can make a significant difference in creating a dark, cave-like atmosphere conducive to deep sleep.

HACK 29- Importance of a Good Mattress

Investing in a good mattress is like investing in a good pair of shoes; it's essential for support and comfort. The right mattress can be the difference between waking up feeling rejuvenated or with aches and pains that last throughout the day.

Firstly, consider the age of your mattress. Most mattresses have a life expectancy of about 8-10 years. If yours is older, it might be time to start looking for a replacement. When choosing a new mattress, personal preference should play a significant role, but there are several key factors to consider:

Firmness:

This should be chosen based on your usual sleep position. Side sleepers generally require a softer mattress to cushion shoulders and hips, back sleepers need medium firmness for lower back support, and stomach sleepers benefit from a firmer mattress to keep the spine aligned.

Material:

Memory foam mattresses adapt to your body shape and reduce

pressure points, but they can retain heat. In contrast, innerspring or hybrid mattresses might offer a cooler sleep with more bounce.

Trial Period:

Many companies now offer a trial period for mattresses, allowing you to sleep on the mattress for several nights before making a commitment. This can be a great way to ensure the mattress suits your needs without risk.

HACK 30- Reducing Blue Light Exposure

In the era of smartphones and screens, blue light exposure has become a major concern, especially in the hours leading up to bedtime. Blue light inhibits the production of melatonin, the hormone that tells our bodies it's time to sleep, thus delaying sleep onset and reducing sleep quality.

Screen Time:

Try to limit exposure to screens at least an hour before bed. If you need to use your devices, most now come with settings that reduce blue light emissions after sunset. Apps that filter blue light can also be installed on devices without this feature.

Light Bulbs:

Consider replacing bright, blue-light-heavy bulbs in your

bedroom with those that emit warmer tones. Bulbs that mimic natural sunlight are best used in areas where you need alertness and concentration, not in spaces intended for relaxation.

Glasses:

If screen use before bed is unavoidable, blue light blocking glasses can be a practical investment. These glasses are designed to filter out blue light and can help minimize its impact on your sleep cycle.

Creating a sleep sanctuary is essentially about minimizing the obstacles to good sleep. By optimizing your bedroom environment, investing in a supportive mattress, and managing blue light exposure, you can transform your bedroom into a space that significantly enhances the quality of your rest. Remember, sleep is not just a biological necessity but a luxurious retreat for your body and mind. Treat it with the care it deserves, and you'll reap the benefits across all areas of your life.

Pre-Sleep Rituals

In the quest for a night of rejuvenating sleep, the rituals you engage in before hitting the pillow play a crucial role. Think of them as a decompression phase, a necessary process to transition your body and mind from the day's hustle into a state of restful repose. Here, we'll explore effective pre-sleep rituals that can dramatically enhance your sleep quality.

HACK 31- Winding Down Routine

Establishing a winding down routine is akin to setting the stage for a grand performance, which in this case, is a deep, restful sleep. About an hour before bed, start by dimming the lights in your living space. Bright lights can trick your mind into thinking it's still daylight, thereby delaying the production of melatonin, the sleep hormone.

Next, engage in calming activities that signal to your body it's time to slow down. This could be reading a book, listening to soft music, or doing some gentle yoga stretches. The key is consistency; performing the same activities in the same order every night can reinforce the body's sleep-wake cycle.

Journaling is another powerful tool in your winding down arsenal. Spend a few minutes reflecting on the day or jotting down what you're grateful for. This practice not only helps in reducing stress but also clears your mind, making it easier to drift off to sleep.

Avoid engaging with electronic devices; their screens emit blue light which can interfere with your ability to fall asleep. If you must use them, consider setting a filter to block blue light or wearing glasses that can offset its effects.

HACK 32- Herbal Teas

Incorporating herbal teas into your nighttime routine can be a game changer. These are not just beverages but ancient remedies that have calmed minds and soothed spirits for centuries. Chamomile tea is a popular choice known for its calming properties that can encourage sleep. Its mild sedative effects can help you feel sleepy and are perfect for those who prefer a natural approach to better sleep.

Valerian root tea is another potent brew worth trying. Some studies suggest that it can improve the speed at which you fall asleep and the quality of that sleep. Its earthy taste might take some getting used to, but the sleep-promoting benefits might just be worth it.

Lavender tea, with its delightful aroma, also makes a great bedtime companion. It's renowned not only for its ability to enhance sleep quality but also for reducing anxiety and relaxing the nerves.

When choosing your night-time tea, ensure its caffeine-free. The last thing you want is a stimulant coursing through your veins when you are trying to calm down. Steep it in hot water for a few minutes, and as you sip slowly, let its warmth and flavors signal to your body that it's time to wind down.

HACK 33- Avoiding Stimulants

It might seem obvious, but stimulants are the arch-nemesis of sleep. Caffeine and nicotine are the main culprits here, notorious for their ability to delay the timing of your sleep and reduce its quality. It's wise to avoid coffee, certain teas, chocolate, and cigarettes late in the day or even in the evening. Remember, caffeine can stay elevated in your blood for 6-8 hours. Even if you don't think caffeine affects you much, it could be silently disrupting your sleep patterns.

Beyond chemicals, stimulating activities can also keep you awake. Intense exercise, engaging work, or emotionally charged conversations late in the evening can rev up your nervous system, making it difficult to wind down. Try to schedule these activities earlier in the day or at least three hours before bedtime.

Alcohol, while often considered a sedative, is particularly sneaky. It might help you fall asleep faster but it dramatically reduces the quality of your sleep, particularly during the second half of the night. This can leave you feeling groggy and unrefreshed come morning. If you enjoy an evening drink, aim to consume it earlier in the evening and limit yourself to one or two.

In conclusion, your pre-sleep rituals can be the cornerstone of good sleep hygiene. By winding down properly, sipping on a soothing herbal tea, and steering clear of stimulants, you're setting yourself up for a night of deep, restorative sleep.

Remember, the key is consistency and mindfulness. By taking control of your bedtime routine, you're not just improving your nights but also every waking moment thereafter.

Sleep Schedules

HACK 34- Consistency in Sleep Times

One secret weapon for optimizing your sleep that often flies under the radar is the art of maintaining consistent sleep times. Think of your body as a finely-tuned orchestra; every instrument needs to start playing at the right moment to create a harmonious performance. Similarly, your body thrives on rhythm—especially when it comes to sleep.

Setting a regular bedtime and wake-up time trains your body's internal clock, or circadian rhythm, to expect rest at certain hours. This conditioning can significantly enhance the quality of your sleep. When you go to bed and wake up at the same time every day, your body becomes accustomed to this routine. As a result, you might find yourself naturally feeling sleepy as bedtime approaches and waking up more refreshed in the morning, often even without the need of an alarm.

It might seem tough to stick to these times every day, especially on weekends or days off, but the payoff is worth it. You can start by setting a realistic bedtime that fits your daily schedule. From there, ensure you're giving yourself enough time to sleep by aiming for the recommended 7-9 hours per night. Gradually, your body will adapt to this schedule, and you'll notice fewer instances of tossing and turning, and more of slipping effortlessly into dreamland.

HACK 35- Power of Napping

While napping isn't a replacement for a good night's sleep, it can certainly complement it, especially on days when you haven't caught enough Zs. A short nap of 20-30 minutes can help to improve mood, alertness, and performance. However, there's a knack to incorporating napping into your life without disrupting your nightly sleep patterns.

Timing is crucial when it comes to napping. Ideally, a nap should be taken early in the afternoon, post-lunch and before 3 PM. This timing works well as it falls during the post-lunch energy dip and is early enough not to interfere with your evening sleep onset. The length of the nap also plays a critical role. Limiting your nap to 20-30 minutes can prevent you from entering deeper stages of sleep, making it easier to wake up feeling refreshed rather than groggy.

For many, napping might seem like a luxury. However, even a brief rest can be a highly effective tool for those who are able to integrate it into their daily routine. It's worth experimenting with napping to see how it affects your energy levels and overall alertness. Remember, the goal is not to extend sleep but to complement the quality of your nightly rest.

HACK 36- Using Sleep Cycles

Understanding sleep cycles can be a game-changer in how you approach your sleep. Sleep is composed of several cycles, each lasting about 90 to 110 minutes. Each cycle includes stages of both non-REM and REM sleep, which are crucial for various functions such as memory consolidation and muscle repair.

To wake up feeling invigorated rather than exhausted, timing your sleep to coincide with the completion of full sleep cycles is key. Waking up in the middle of a sleep cycle can leave you feeling groggy and disoriented. In contrast, waking up between cycles, when your sleep is lightest, can help you start your day with more energy.

A practical way to apply this knowledge is by planning your sleep schedule around these cycles. For example, if you aim to sleep for 7.5 hours, you're looking at fitting in five complete sleep cycles (7.5 divided by 1.5 hours per cycle). Adjusting your bedtime or wake-up time slightly can help you align this schedule more closely with your natural sleep cycles.

Many find technology helpful in tracking their sleep cycles, using smartwatches and apps that analyze sleep patterns and suggest optimal sleep schedules. While technology can be useful, it's also important to listen to your body. Paying attention to when you naturally wake up without an alarm can give you insights into your personal sleep cycle duration.

Incorporating knowledge about sleep cycles into your routine isn't about strict adherence to numbers but rather about understanding your body's natural rhythms and using that knowledge to enhance the restorative power of sleep.

By embracing these principles—consistency in sleep times, the strategic use of napping, and aligning with your natural sleep cycles—you can transform not only how you sleep but also how you function and feel during your waking hours. Each component works synergistically, creating a robust framework that supports and enhances your overall health and well-being. By optimizing your sleep schedule, you're not just investing in better nights; you're setting the stage for more vibrant, energetic days.

RECAP AND ACTION ITEMS ON THE 9 OPTIMISE YOUR SLEEP HACKS

By now, you've armed yourself with crucial strategies to unlock the full potential of your slumber. Think of this as a toolkit to enhance every aspect of your sleep, ensuring you wake up refreshed and ready to take on the world every day. Let's quickly recap the key points and jump straight into some actionable steps you can implement tonight.

Firstly, transforming your bedroom into a sleep sanctuary is essential. Ensure your environment is primed for optimal rest by keeping it cool, dark, and quiet. Investing in a good mattress might seem like a hefty upfront cost, but it's a game changer for your body's recovery and overall health. Also, don't forget to minimize your exposure to blue light in the evenings by tweaking the settings on your devices or wearing blue light blocking glasses.

Moving on to your pre-sleep rituals, establishing a winding-down routine is crucial. Whether it's reading, stretching, or practicing mindfulness, find what soothes you and make it a nightly habit. Integrating herbal teas can also be a fantastic way to signal to your body that it's time to wind down. Remember, avoiding stimulants like caffeine and nicotine close to bedtime will prevent them from sabotaging your sleep quality.

Lastly, adhering to a consistent sleep schedule will regulate your body's internal clock, while understanding the power of napping can boost your alertness and productivity without compromising your nightly rest. Tailoring your sleep to align with natural cycles can further enhance the quality of rest you achieve.

ACTION STEPS TO TAKE TONIGHT:

Audit Your Sleep Environment:

Assess your current bedroom setup and make adjustments where necessary. Aim for a cool, dark, and quiet environment

Establish a Pre-Sleep Ritual:

Tonight, select a relaxing activity to do 30 minutes before bed. Whether it's reading a book or sipping on a cup of chamomile tea, make it a consistent part of your routine

Set a Consistent Bedtime:

Choose a realistic time to go to bed and wake up, and stick to it—even on weekends

Experiment with Napping:

If you feel an afternoon slump, try a short, 20-minute nap to refresh your mind. Observe how it affects your energy levels and night-time sleep quality.

Implementing these steps will set you on a path towards improved sleep and, consequently, a healthier, more vibrant life. Remember, the journey to better sleep doesn't happen overnight. Be patient with yourself, make adjustments as needed, and most importantly, listen to your body. It knows what it needs; sometimes, we just need to pay better attention.

5

HYDRATION HACKS

"Water is the driving force of all nature." - Leonardo da Vinci

Understanding Hydration

HACK 37- Benefits of Staying Hydrated

Hydration is not just about quenching your thirst; it's a cornerstone of wellness that affects virtually every function within your body. You might already know that about 60% of your body is water, but have you ever paused to think about the implications of this fact? Water is essential for your organs to function properly, it keeps your skin healthy and glowing, and it even influences your energy levels and cognitive functions.

First off, staying well-hydrated helps in maintaining your

body's fluid balance, which aids in transportation of nutrients, digestion, and regulation of body temperature. When you drink sufficient water, your body is better equipped to break down food, absorb nutrients and eliminate waste products in an efficient manner, all of which are vital processes for optimal health.

Moreover, proper hydration can enhance your physical performance. Dehydration can lead to decreased strength, reduced endurance, increased fatigue, and an elevated risk of cramps, which means staying hydrated is essential for anyone who engages in physical activity, no matter the intensity level.

Mental clarity is another significant benefit. Even mild dehydration can impair attention span, memory, and motor skills. By keeping yourself hydrated, you can help ensure that your brain is operating at its best. Think of water as the fuel your brain needs to fire on all cylinders.

Lastly, water plays a crucial role in regulating your body's cooling system. Sweating helps to keep your body cool, but if you're not hydrated, your body can't produce enough sweat, and you might overheat. This is particularly critical during intense exercise or hot weather.

HACK 38- Signs of Dehydration

Recognizing the signs of dehydration is crucial because the sensations of thirst can often be misinterpreted or go unnoticed until dehydration becomes severe. Common signs include dry mouth, tiredness, and less frequent urination than usual. If your urine is dark yellow, this is a clear indicator that you need to drink more water.

Other signs might be less obvious but equally important to recognize. These include dry, flushed skin, headaches, and dizziness. In severe cases, a lack of proper hydration can lead to heat injuries such as heat stroke, especially in hot weather.

One surprising indicator of dehydration is bad breath. Saliva has antibacterial properties, and without enough of it, bacteria can thrive, leading to bad breath. Moreover, feeling unusually hungry can also be a sign. Sometimes, the body confuses thirst with hunger. Drinking a glass of water before reaching for a snack can help you determine if you're truly hungry or just dehydrated.

HACK 39- Daily Water Intake Calculation

So how much water should you be drinking? The old adage of eight glasses a day is a good starting point, but it oversimplifies the hydration needs that can vary greatly depending on age, weight, climate, and activity level.

A more tailored approach is to drink between 1-1.5 milliliters of water per calorie of energy expended. For the average adult consuming about 2 000 calories per day, that translates roughly to 2 to 3 liters a day. However, if you're particularly active, you might need more.

A practical way to calculate your ideal water intake is to take your weight in kilograms and multiply it by 0.033. So, if you weigh60 kilograms, you should be aiming for about 2 liters of water a day. Remember, this is a baseline and needs to be adjusted according to your daily activities and the climate you live in.

To put it into perspective, if you exercise frequently, you lose water not just in the form of sweat but also through exhaled breath. Therefore, it's essential to increase your water intake on days when you are more physically active or when the weather is particularly hot.

Moreover, it's not just about water. All fluids count towards your daily hydration needs, although water should ideally be your primary source because it's free from calories, additives, and sugars that can be found in other beverages. However, foods with high water content, such as fruits and vegetables, also contribute significantly to your daily water intake.

Hydration isn't just a health issue; it's a quality of life issue. Staying adequately hydrated helps you to function at your best, both physically and mentally. Start treating your hydration as a priority, and you'll notice improvements not just in your health, but in your overall life satisfaction. Remember, water is not just life-sustaining; it's life-enhancing.

Fun with Fluids

Drinking enough water every day is a non-negotiable for good health, but let's face it—constantly sipping plain water can feel a bit like a chore. So, how about jazzing things up a bit? Infusing some fun into your hydration routine not only makes it more enjoyable but can also tempt you to drink more than you usually would. Here are some creative ways to stay hydrated without relying solely on plain water.

HACK 40- Infused Water Ideas

Infused water, also known as detox water, has been a favorite for health enthusiasts and influencers alike—and for good reason. Not only is it incredibly easy to make, but it also offers a refreshing twist to your hydration habits with minimal calories. The process involves steeping fruits, vegetables, and herbs in cold water, which allows their flavors and nutrients to blend beautifully with the liquid.

Begin with the basics like cucumber and mint, which not only tastes fresh but also aids in digestion and adds a gentle boost to your metabolism. Simply slice half a cucumber and tear a handful of mint leaves, add them to a jug of water and let them infuse overnight in the fridge.

For something a little zestier, try lemon and ginger. This combo not only perks up your water but also packs it with vitamin C and anti-inflammatory benefits. Thinly slice a lemon and some ginger root, and let them sit in water for a few hours or overnight to fully release their flavors.

Berries are another fantastic option for infused water. Try a mix of strawberries and blueberries for a sweet, tangy twist that's loaded with antioxidants. Just chop the strawberries and toss them into a pitcher of water with a handful of whole blueberries. Give them a few hours to infuse, and you've got a delicious drink that looks as good as it tastes.

Get creative and experiment with different combinations to find what you enjoy most. The possibilities are endless!

HACK 41- Herbal Teas

Moving beyond water, herbal teas offer a fantastic way to stay hydrated while also providing a plethora of health benefits. Unlike their caffeinated counterparts, herbal teas are hydrating and can be a calming ritual to incorporate into your day.

Chamomile tea is a popular choice for its soothing properties, making it a perfect evening drink that can help you unwind before bed. It's not only good for relaxation but also aids in digestion.

Peppermint tea is another great option, especially if you're prone to digestive troubles. It has a refreshing taste and is known to relieve symptoms of bloating, cramps, and nausea.

For a more invigorating option, try ginger tea. Known for its anti-inflammatory properties, it can help reduce pain and improve digestion. A slice of lemon added to your ginger tea can enhance its flavor and up its vitamin C content, giving your immune system a little boost.

Remember, you can enjoy these teas hot or cold, making them a versatile choice year-round. If you prefer a sweet touch, consider adding a teaspoon of honey or a few drops of stevia rather than refined sugar to keep things healthier.

HACK 42- Hydrating Foods

Last but certainly not least, let's talk about hydrating foods. Yes, you can eat your water—quite literally! Incorporating water-rich foods into your diet is an excellent way to boost your hydration.

Cucumbers top the list with about 96% water content, making them a super hydrator. Add them to your salads, munch on them as a snack, or blend them into a smoothie.

Watermelons are not just a summer favorite, but they are also made up of over 90% water. Plus, they're rich in vitamins A and C, making them a nutritious choice for a hydrating snack.

Oranges, strawberries, and grapefruits are also packed with juice and are great for hydration. These fruits offer the added bonus of vitamin C, which helps in boosting your immune system.

Don't forget about soups and broths. These are especially comforting in cooler weather and can be a significant source of hydration. Opt for broth-based soups rather than creamy ones to keep it light and hydrating.

Incorporating these foods into your daily diet can significantly contribute to your overall fluid intake without having to chug water constantly.

By exploring these options—infused waters, herbal teas, and hydrating foods—you can make staying hydrated an enjoyable part of your day. These choices not only improve how you feel but also add a splash of variety and flavor to your routine, making it easier to drink those essential fluids. So go ahead, have fun with your fluids and keep sipping your way to better health.

Hydration Monitoring

HACK 43- Tracking Your Intake

The first step in really getting a grip on your hydration is to know exactly how much you're drinking. It sounds simple, but tracking your daily water intake can be an eye-opening experience. Most people think they're drinking enough fluids, but when they start to record every glass, they often find they're falling short.

So, how do you track your intake? You could go old school with a pen and paper, jotting down each drink as you have it. However, in the spirit of efficiency and convenience, using a daily planner or a dedicated section in your journal can integrate this habit into your routine seamlessly. Every time you drink a glass of water or any other liquid, make a note of the amount. To make this even simpler, keep a standard-sized water bottle on hand; knowing the volume it holds can help you easily tally your total intake without too much fuss.

A visual method that many find helpful is the use of a hydration tracking chart. You can create one with columns for each day and rows for each glass of water. Every time you finish a drink, fill in a box. This gives you a clear, visual representation of your hydration over the week, making it easier to spot patterns and adjust accordingly.

Remember, the goal here isn't just to meet a quota; it's to understand your body's needs and how they vary depending on activity level, the weather, and your health. By keeping track of what you drink, you're taking a proactive step towards better hydration, which can lead to improved energy levels, better skin health, and overall enhanced well-being.

HACK 44- Setting Reminders

Life gets busy, and it's easy to forget to pause and take a sip of water. This is where setting reminders can be a game-changer. In our digital age, there are countless ways to nudge yourself to drink more water. You might set alarms on your phone or use a smartwatch that buzzes at regular intervals as a reminder to take a drink.

If you're a fan of technology, you can integrate these reminders into your existing routine. For instance, set a reminder to drink water every hour or after certain activities like after a meeting, post-workout, or right before you leave for work. You could also link your reminders with daily tasks; for example, drink a glass of water before each meal. This not only helps you stay hydrated but also aids in digestion.

For those who prefer a less tech-heavy approach, simple strategies like keeping a water bottle visibly on your desk or carrying one in your bag can serve as a physical reminder. Each time you see your bottle, take it as a cue to hydrate. Alternatively, you could position glasses of water in different rooms around your home. This method ensures that wherever you go, a reminder to drink water is never too far away.

HACK 45- Using Apps

There's an app for almost everything these days, and hydration is no exception. Several apps are designed to help you track and improve your water intake. These apps often come with customizable features, such as setting your daily water intake goals, logging different types of drinks, and providing detailed statistics about your hydration over time.

Apps like 'Daily Water Tracker Reminder' and 'Hydro Coach' allow you to input your weight, age, and activity level to calculate your optimal daily water intake. They send timely reminders throughout the day and can adjust the frequency of these reminders based on your past intake or even the local weather conditions—more water might be nudged on hotter days.

Furthermore, these apps often incorporate gamification elements to make the process of staying hydrated more engaging. You might earn badges or achieve milestones, which can be particularly motivating if you're the type of person who enjoys a challenge or thrives on positive reinforcement.

Using an app can also help you visualize your progress. Many hydration apps provide graphs and analytics, so you can see your hydration levels over time and understand how your intake affects your mood, energy levels, and physical performance. This feedback loop can be incredibly valuable in making sustained changes to your habits.

Tracking, reminding, and utilizing tools are all about making hydration a conscious part of your day. By monitoring your intake, setting thoughtful reminders, and perhaps harnessing the power of apps, you're equipping yourself with the knowledge and habits that lead to better health and vitality. Remember, every sip counts towards a more energized and vibrant you.

RECAP AND ACTION ITEMS ON THE 9 HYDRATION HACKS

Hydration might seem like a basic element of health, but as you've discovered, it's a powerhouse of an ally in your quest for vitality and wellness. We've unpacked the essentials of staying adequately hydrated, explored some creative avenues to make hydration enjoyable, and equipped you with tools to monitor your water intake effectively. Now, let's put that knowledge into action.

Firstly, take a moment to appreciate the profound benefits hydration brings to your body, from boosting your energy levels to enhancing skin health. With this understanding, make a personal commitment to honor your body's hydration needs.

Begin by calculating your daily water intake using the guidelines provided. Remember, factors like your activity level, climate, and health conditions can influence how much water you should be drinking. Make it a morning ritual to set your hydration goal for the day.

Next, infuse some fun into your fluids. Start tomorrow by trying one of the infused water recipes — perhaps a refreshing cucumber and mint or a zesty lemon and ginger. Experiment with different combinations each week to keep things exciting and flavorful. Don't forget about herbal teas; they are a fantastic way to vary your intake while reaping herbal benefits. Peppermint, chamomile, or hibiscus can be delightful choices that both hydrate and relax you.

Incorporate hydrating foods into your diet regularly. Foods like cucumber, celery, and watermelon are not only packed with water but also vitamins and minerals, making them a double win for your health. Aim to include at least one hydrating food in every meal.

Finally, leverage technology to keep your hydration on track. Use an app to log your daily water intake, which can help you see patterns and make necessary adjustments. Set reminders on your phone or smartwatch to take a hydration break, which can be particularly useful if you have a busy schedule or tend to forget to drink water.

By making these small, manageable changes, you empower yourself to maintain optimal hydration levels consistently. This simple yet effective strategy will support your overall health and enhance your life's quality, allowing you to live better, longer, and more fulfilled. Embrace the fluidity of life by keeping your hydration in check—it's a small step towards monumental health benefits.

6

MOVEMENT FOR LONGEVITY

"Movement is a medicine for creating change in a person's physical, emotional, and mental states." - Carol Welch

Daily Movement Goals

In the bustling rhythm of modern life, finding time for exercise can often fall by the wayside. Yet, the secret to boosting your health and enhancing your longevity might just lie in setting daily movement goals. Let's break this down into manageable parts: Setting Realistic Goals, Variety in Exercise, and the Importance of Stretching.

HACK 46- Setting Realistic Goals

The journey to a healthier you begins with setting achievable daily movement goals. It's about crafting a plan that aligns with your current fitness level and lifestyle, rather than adopting an all-or-nothing approach. Start by asking yourself what is realistically manageable for you right now, not what you think you should be doing based on fitness trends or societal pressures.

For many, a good starting point might be as simple as a daily 10-minute walk. It's low impact, requires no special equipment, and can be done almost anywhere. The key here is consistency over intensity. As you build your routine, these small increments of regular activity can significantly contribute to your overall health and energy levels.

Remember, the aim here is not to train for an ultramarathon (unless that's your thing!), but to incorporate more movement into your everyday life. Gradually increase the duration or intensity of your activities as you become more comfortable and confident. This could mean increasing your walk to 20 minutes, or introducing a light jog or cycle a few days a week.

HACK 47- Variety in Exercise

Once you have established a routine, introducing a variety of exercises can be beneficial not just for your body, but also for your mind. Engaging in different types of activities can prevent boredom, reduce the risk of overuse injuries, and ensure that all muscle groups are being worked.

Think about including a mix of cardiovascular exercises, strength training, and perhaps something for flexibility like yoga or Pilates. Each type of exercise offers distinct benefits. Cardiovascular activities like running, swimming, or cycling are great for improving heart and lung health, while strength training such as lifting weights or body-weight exercises helps to build muscle and strengthen bones.

To keep things exciting, why not try something new every few weeks? This could be anything from a dance class to a rock climbing session. The novelty can be incredibly motivating and can help you discover new passions while keeping your fitness journey fresh and engaging.

HACK 48- Importance of Stretching

Often overlooked, stretching is a crucial component of any fitness regime and plays a vital role in improving flexibility and range of motion. Regular stretching can also aid in injury prevention and contribute to better posture, which is particularly important if you find yourself sitting at a desk for long periods.

Incorporate stretching into your daily routine by setting aside time either before or after your main exercise session. Alternatively, consider it as a calming activity to wind down your day. Focus on major muscle groups such as your legs, hips, back, and shoulders. Hold each stretch for about 20-30 seconds and avoid bouncing, which can cause muscle strain.

Dynamic stretches, which involve moving as you stretch, are great before a workout to help warm up the body. These might include leg swings or arm circles, which prepare your body for physical activity by increasing blood flow to the muscles. Post-exercise, opt for static stretches where you hold a position for a longer period. This helps to cool down the body and can reduce muscle stiffness and soreness.

Setting daily movement goals is not about pushing yourself to the extreme but about integrating more activity into your life in a fun and sustainable way. Whether it's opting for the stairs instead of the elevator, going for a walk during your lunch break, or stretching while watching TV, every little bit adds up. Remember, the goal is to enhance your health and energy, paving the way for a more active, fulfilled life. By setting realistic goals, embracing variety, and not neglecting stretching, you lay down the foundations for a lifetime of improved wellbeing and vitality.

Fun Fitness

When it comes to staying active and keeping fit, the magic often lies in how much fun you can have while doing it. If you dread the thought of another run on the treadmill or can't face lifting another weight, it might be time to inject some joy back into your fitness regime. Let's dive into some exciting ways you can stay in shape, without it feeling like a chore.

HACK 49- Dance Workouts

There's a reason why dance floors are always packed at weddings and parties: dancing is exhilarating. It's not only a blast but also an excellent workout. Dance workouts can catapult your fitness to new heights, all while you're moving to the beat of your favorite tunes.

Imagine combining the thrill of dancing with the structure of a workout. Classes like Zumba, Hip-Hop aerobics, or even ballet-inspired fitness programs are not just about burning calories—they are about letting loose and expressing yourself. These sessions are typically designed to cater to all fitness levels, ensuring that everyone from beginners to seasoned dancers can keep up and have fun.

The beauty of dance workouts lies in their versatility. They improve your cardiovascular health, tone your muscles, and enhance your coordination and balance. Each routine can be a full-body workout that keeps the boredom at bay. And the best part? You might be so engrossed in learning new moves that you forget you're working out at all. So, lace up those dancing shoes and let your living room, local gym, or any space you find yourself in become your dance floor.

HACK 50- Outdoor Activities

Stepping outside can do more than just give you a change of scenery. Engaging in outdoor activities taps into the adventurous side of fitness, making it an exciting and effective way to enhance your physical and mental health.

Whether it's hiking through winding trails, cycling in the park, kayaking on a lake, or simply taking a brisk walk in your neighborhood, the great outdoors offers a plethora of options to keep fit. The natural terrain provides a natural resistance and varied intensity, which can help to improve your endurance and strength more effectively than many indoor exercises.

Moreover, outdoor activities can be a fantastic social activity. Join a walking group, a cycling club, or an outdoor fitness class. Not only will you benefit from the physical exercise, but the social interaction can boost your mood and motivation levels.

Don't underestimate the mental health benefits either. Being in nature reduces stress, enhances mood, and improves overall wellbeing. So, whether it's sunny, slightly overcast, or even a bit chilly, dressing appropriately and getting outside can add a refreshing element to your fitness regimen.

HACK 51 - Group Sports

Remember the sheer joy of playing sports at school or in the park as a child? Recapturing that feeling as an adult isn't just good for your nostalgia; it's great for your health. Group sports such as football, basketball, volleyball, or even less conventional sports like ultimate frisbee or tag rugby can be exhilarating ways to stay fit.

Playing sports in a team setting not only pushes you physically but also challenges you mentally. The strategic thinking, quick decision-making, and mental alertness required in these sports provide a cerebral workout that many solo fitness routines can't match.

One of the biggest advantages of engaging in group sports is the accountability it offers. It's easier to bail on a solo workout than on a team that counts on your participation. Plus, the social aspect of meeting with a team regularly can enhance your commitment to fitness and provide a supportive environment that encourages persistence.

Furthermore, group sports can be tailored to your fitness level and interest. Most community leagues offer various tiers from recreational to competitive. This means you can find the right fit for your skill level and enjoy the game without feeling over-challenged or underwhelmed.

Incorporating fun into your fitness routine isn't just a way to alleviate the monotony of more traditional exercises; it's essential for long-term adherence and success. By exploring dance workouts, embracing the great outdoors, or joining a sports team, you transform exercise from a dreaded duty into a delightful diversion. And who knows? You might just find your new passion while you're at it.

Age-Defying Exercises

HACK 52- Strength Training

Contrary to popular myth, strength training isn't just for the young or aspiring bodybuilders; it's a golden ticket to aging gracefully. Incorporating strength training into your routine can significantly enhance muscle mass, which naturally begins to decline from your 30s onwards. This isn't just about bulking up; it's about sustaining the muscle needed for everyday activities — carrying groceries, climbing stairs, or playing with your grandchildren.

Start with basics like squats, push-ups, and lunges. These exercises use your body weight to build strength, making them easily accessible regardless of whether you're at home or can hit the gym. The key is consistency rather than intensity. Aim for two to three sessions per week, focusing on major muscle groups — legs, hips, back, abdomen, chest, shoulders, and arms. The use of resistance bands, dumbbells, or even cans of beans can add variety and challenge as you progress.

Remember, the goal here isn't to lift the heaviest weights possible but to maintain a level of fitness that keeps your body strong and functional. If you're unsure about techniques, consider a session or two with a personal trainer. They can provide guidance tailored specifically to your needs, ensuring you perform exercises correctly and safely.

HACK 53- Balance Exercises

As we age, our balance can deteriorate, which increases the risk of falls. However, with regular balance exercises, you can enhance your stability and coordination, making falls less likely. Balance training is all about teaching your body and brain to work together more effectively, ensuring you can react swiftly if you start to trip or wobble.

Start simple with exercises like standing on one foot, which you can do almost anytime, anywhere. For an added challenge, try it with your eyes closed or while performing upper body movements. Tai chi, often referred to as "meditation in motion," is another excellent method for improving balance. This gentle form of martial arts involves slow, controlled movements that can help strengthen your body's stabilizing muscles while calming your mind.

Incorporate balance workouts into your routine at least three days a week. These exercises can be quick and straightforward; even a few minutes can be beneficial. As you progress, integrate dynamic movements like walking heel-to-toe or using a balance board. Activities like yoga can also be incredibly effective in improving your balance and overall flexibility.

HACK 54- Flexibility Workouts

The importance of flexibility cannot be overstated, especially as you age. Increasing your flexibility can drastically reduce your risk of injuries, relieve joint pain, and improve your range of motion. This means better posture, less back pain, and easier movement in daily tasks.

Yoga is a fantastic way to improve flexibility. It stretches all parts of the body and can be adapted to all levels of fitness and experience. Start with basic poses like the cat-cow for spinal flexibility, the pigeon pose for hip opening, and the forward bend for hamstring stretching. Yoga not only helps with flexibility but also incorporates breathing exercises and meditation that can reduce stress and enhance mental clarity.

Don't overlook the importance of a simple stretch, either. Regular stretching routines, especially after other forms of exercise, can help maintain the elasticity of your muscles and tendons. Focus on major muscle groups and hold stretches for about 30 seconds. Remember, stretching should feel good; if you feel any pain, you've pushed too far.

Including flexibility workouts in your regimen at least three to four times a week will help keep your body limber and pain-free. These sessions don't have to be long; even 10 to 15 minutes can make a significant difference. As with any exercise, the key is regularity; make stretching a habit, and your future self will thank you.

By integrating these age-defying exercises into your fitness routine, you are not just investing in your current health but are setting the stage for a vigorous, active future. Strength training, balance exercises, and flexibility workouts are your allies in maintaining independence and vitality as you age. So, take the challenge, embrace these practices, and transform your later years into some of your best yet.

RECAP AND ACTION ITEMS ON THE 9 MOVEMENT FOR LONGEVITY HACKS

Congratulations on completing this chapter on Movement for Longevity! By now, you should feel equipped with essential strategies to keep your body moving effectively for years to come. Let's take a quick look back and set some actionable steps to integrate these insights into your daily life.

Firstly, we discussed the importance of setting realistic goals in your exercise regimen. Tailoring your daily movement to fit your current fitness level and lifestyle ensures sustainability and reduces the risk of burnout or injury. Start by setting small, achievable goals that gradually build in intensity and duration. Whether it's a 15-minute walk after dinner or a set of gentle stretches each morning, the key is consistency.

Variety in your exercise routine not only keeps things interesting but also ensures that all muscle groups get their fair share of attention. Mix things up! If you've enjoyed a brisk walk today, consider a light yoga session tomorrow, followed by some cycling or swimming later in the week. This approach helps to work different muscles and improves overall body function.

Stretching, often overlooked, is crucial for maintaining flexibility and preventing injuries. Incorporate a short stretching routine into your daily plan, focusing on major muscle groups. This can enhance your performance in other physical activities and increase your range of motion.

Turning to Fun Fitness, remember that exercise doesn't have to be a chore. Dance workouts, outdoor activities, and group sports are fantastic ways to inject some joy into staying active. Choose activities that you enjoy, and you're more likely to stick with them long-term. Whether it's salsa dancing, hiking through nature trails, or joining a local football team, the goal is to have fun while moving your body.

Lastly, embracing age-defying exercises like strength training, balance workouts, and flexibility routines will serve you well as you age. Strength training helps maintain muscle mass and bone density, balance exercises reduce the risk of falls, and flexibility workouts keep your joints supple.

ACTION STEPS:

Set a small, achievable movement goal for tomorrow. It could be anything from a10-minute stretch session to a half-hour walk

Plan a week's worth of activities, ensuring to include a variety of exercises. Perhaps pencil in a dance class, a strength training session, and a balance-focused activity

Identify a fun activity you've never tried before but have always wanted to. Make arrangements to start this within the next month

Invest in a good pair of trainers and comfortable workout attire that will encourage you to stay active

Share your plans with a friend or family member and invite them to join you on this journey. Accountability can be a powerful motivator.

By integrating these practices into your lifestyle, you're not just investing in your longevity; you're enhancing your daily quality of life. Here's to a healthier, more energetic, and fulfilling life ahead!

7

NUTRITION KNOW-HOW

"Let food be thy medicine and medicine be thy food." - *Hippocrates*

Fundamentals of Balanced Eating

Eating right isn't just about shedding a few pounds or prepping for that upcoming holiday; it's about setting the stage for a fuller, more vibrant life. Let's dive straight into the core of balanced eating, ensuring you're not just fueled but also flourishing through your everyday.

HACK 55- Macronutrients and Micronutrients

Understanding the basics of what you consume can transform your approach to food. Let's start with macronutrients - those big players that provide you with energy (calories). They are carbohydrates, proteins, and fats. Each one has its unique role in your body and, contrary to popular belief, all are essential.

Carbohydrates are your body's main energy source. They're not just about bread and pasta; fruits, vegetables, and legumes are fantastic sources too. Proteins are vital for muscle repair and growth, impacting everything from your physical strength to your metabolic rate. They come power-packed in foods like chicken, tofu, and lentils. Then, there's fat – often villainized but crucial for your body. Fats help absorb vitamins and provide essential fatty acids. Avocado, nuts, and oily fish are excellent sources.

Now, for micronutrients - these are the vitamins and minerals that support myriad body functions from bone health to immune system strength. While they don't provide energy like macros, their role in your health orchestra is just as crucial. Iron, found in lean meats and spinach, is key for blood health, while vitamin C from oranges and strawberries boosts your immune system.

A balanced diet means getting the right ratio of these nutrients. The "perfect plate" might look like half filled with vegetables (micronutrients galore), a quarter with lean proteins, and a quarter with complex carbs, topped off with a sprinkle of healthy fats.

HACK 56- Reading Food Labels

Navigating food labels can sometimes feel like cracking a code. But once you know what to look for, it's a breeze – and it can make a huge difference in your eating habits. Start with the basics: serving size. This is the first thing you should look at because all the nutritional info you're about to read pertains to this specific amount of food.

Next up, calories. Remember, not all calories are created equal, so pair this information with what you know about macros and micros. For a healthier choice, look beyond calories; check the sources. Is the fat coming from olive oil or butter? Are the sugars added, or are they coming from fruits?

The ingredients list is your best friend. Ingredients are listed in order of quantity, so if sugar or something unpronounceable is near the top, you might want to reconsider your choice. Be on the lookout for hidden sugars and fats, often disguised under different names (like "corn syrup" or "hydrogenated oils").

Lastly, pay attention to the fiber and protein content, especially if you're trying to feel fuller for longer. These can turn a snack from a quick fix into a sustaining food choice.

HACK 57- Portion Control

In a world of super-sized meals and heaping plates, portion control is your secret weapon. It's not just about reducing the amount of food you eat but understanding how much food your body actually needs.

A handy method is using your hand as a guide: a fist-sized serving of carbs, a palm-sized portion of protein, and a thumb-sized serving of healthy fats. Vegetables? Load them up – the more, the merrier (within reason, of course).

Remember, eating directly from a large packet or container can lead to overeating. Try serving yourself a specific amount on a plate or in a bowl rather than eating mindlessly. And during meals, it helps to eat slowly. It takes about20 minutes for your brain to register that you're full, so give it time to catch up to your stomach.

Portion control isn't just about eating less; it's about eating right. It's knowing that sometimes, a smaller, nutrient-rich meal can fuel you better than a large, nutrient-poor one. This approach not only helps in maintaining a healthy weight but also in enhancing your overall relationship with food.

By grasping these fundamentals of balanced eating, you're not just feeding yourself; you're preparing for a lifetime of energy and vitality. So, take this knowledge, apply it day by day, and watch as your body thanks you in countless ways.

Superfoods and Their Superpowers

HACK 58- Berries

Let's kick off with nature's colorful jewels: berries. Bursting with vitamins, antioxidants, and fiber, these little powerhouses are your new best mates for boosting health. Think of blueberries, strawberries, raspberries, and blackberries as your go-to arsenal for a vibrant life.

First up, blueberries are often touted as the king of antioxidant foods. They're loaded with Vitamin C and Vitamin K. The antioxidants in blueberries, particularly anthocyanins, help fight oxidative stress in your body and can boost your immune system. Regular consumption might also enhance your brain health, reducing the risk of cognitive decline as you age.

Strawberries, on the other hand, are not only juicy and delicious but also a fantastic source of Vitamin C. This vitamin is crucial for the maintenance of skin integrity and immune function. Furthermore, the seeds of strawberries are a good source of dietary fiber.

Raspberries are fiber champions, offering about 8 grams per cup. High fiber content not only aids digestion but can also help you manage your weight by keeping you fuller longer. Plus, these berries are high in manganese, which is essential for bone development and nutrient absorption.

Lastly, blackberries are similar to their berry cousins but stand out with their high Vitamin K content, critical for bone health and wound healing.

To incorporate these into your diet, think beyond just having them as a snack. Sprinkle berries on your morning cereal, blend them into a smoothie, or toss them in a salad for a fresh, sweet kick.

HACK 59- Nuts and Seeds

Nuts and seeds are the unsung heroes in the world of nutrition. They're tiny but mighty sources of essential fats, proteins, vitamins, and minerals. Let's break down why these should be a staple in your pantry.

Almonds, for instance, are incredibly nutrient-rich. They offer a fantastic source of Vitamin E, which is key for maintaining healthy skin and eyes. They're also packed with magnesium, vital for muscle function and sleep regulation.

Walnuts are another superfood star, known particularly for their high levels of omega-3 fatty acids, comparable to those found in fish. These fats are crucial for cognitive function and maintaining heart health. Regular intake of walnuts can help manage cholesterol levels and calm the inflammation storm in your body.

Seeds like chia and flaxseeds are also worth your attention. Chia seeds are full of fiber, omega-3 fatty acids, and several essential minerals. They're incredibly absorbent and develop a gel-like texture when soaked, making them perfect for thickening smoothies or making a 'chia pudding'. Flaxseeds, meanwhile, are a top source of lignans, which have been shown to decrease cancer risk and improve cardiovascular health.

To make the most of these nutritional powerhouses, throw a handful into your yoghurt, blend into smoothies, or bake into muffins. Remember that while nuts and seeds are high in nutrients, they're also calorie-dense, so mindful portioning is key.

HACK 60- Green Leafy Vegetables

The champions of the vegetable aisle—green leafy vegetables. Kale, spinach, and Swiss chard are packed with vitamins, minerals, and fibers yet low in calories. They're your golden ticket to a nutrient-packed diet.

Kale, for example, is not just a trend—it's one of the most nutrient-dense foods on the planet. It's loaded with vitamins A, K, C, and minerals like manganese. Eating kale can help improve bone health, and its high antioxidant content may lower your risk of developing chronic illnesses.

Spinach is another all-star, rich in iron which is vital for creating hemoglobin, a protein needed to deliver oxygen throughout your body. It's also high in vitamin K, vitamin A, vitamin C, and folic acid, a B-vitamin that helps prevent neural tube defects in pregnancies.

Swiss chard has a unique property—it's high in nitrates, which improve muscle oxygenation during exercise. This can enhance your performance and endurance. Like its cousins, it's also high in vitamins A, C, and K.

To use these green giants, sauté them with a bit of olive oil and garlic for a delicious side dish, toss them into a smoothie for a nutrient boost, or add them to soups and stews.

Incorporating berries, nuts, seeds, and green leafy vegetables into your diet isn't just about eating healthily; it's about making smarter food choices that empower your body's natural resilience and vitality. Embrace these superfoods and let their superpowers help you live a healthier, longer life.

Smart Snacking

HACK 61- Healthy Snack Ideas

Let's face it, snacking is inevitable. Whether you're feeling that mid-afternoon slump or need something to tide you over until dinner, reaching for a snack is part of our daily ritual. But here's the kicker: it doesn't have to be a diet disaster. Snacking smart can actually be a strategic part of your nutrition plan, helping you maintain energy levels, control appetite, and even boost overall health.

First up, think protein. This isn't just for gym buffs – protein is a vital macronutrient that helps in tissue repair and provides energy. How about roasted chickpeas? They're crispy, tasty, and you can toss them with any seasoning you fancy – chili powder for a kick, or maybe some rosemary and garlic for a savory treat. Greek yoghurt is another excellent choice. Top it with a sprinkle of chia seeds for a texture twist and a punch of omega-3 fatty acids.

Fruits and vegetables are your friends, too. Ever tried apple slices with almond butter? The combo of sweet and nutty flavors is not only mouth-watering but also packs a nutritional punch. Carrot sticks or bell pepper slices dipped in hummus make another colorful, crunchy option that's full of fiber and protein.

And let's not forget about nuts. A small handful of almonds, walnuts, or Brazil nuts provides a satisfying crunch along with essential fats, proteins, and a range of micronutrients. Just be mindful of portion sizes, as nuts are calorie-dense.

HACK 62- Timing Your Snacks

Timing is everything, especially when it comes to snacking. The goal here is to fuel your body in a way that enhances your energy levels without overloading it just before meal times. A good rule of thumb is to listen to your body and learn to recognize true hunger cues. Are you really hungry, or are you bored, stressed, or thirsty? Keeping hydrated can often curb the urge to snack unnecessarily.

Aim to space your snacks evenly between meals. Mid-morning, think about something rich in fiber like a small oat bar or a piece of fruit to keep you full. This is particularly effective to avoid the lunchtime overeat. For the afternoon, lean towards protein-rich snacks like a boiled egg or a piece of cheese. These will keep you satisfied and prevent the dreaded end-of-day energy crash.

Consider your daily routine and activity level as well. If you're planning a workout, a banana or a small smoothie about 30 to 60 minutes beforehand can provide a quick energy boost. Post-exercise, a little protein can help muscle recovery, so perhaps a few slices of turkey or a protein shake.

HACK 63- Snacks to Avoid

While snacking can be part of a healthy diet, some choices can undermine your best intentions. Here's the scoop on what types of snacks to steer clear of.

Highly processed snacks are the biggest culprits. Yes, those pre-packaged cakes, biscuits, and crisps are convenient, but they're often loaded with sugar, unhealthy fats, and salt – not to mention a host of preservatives and artificial ingredients you probably can't pronounce. These can spike your blood sugar levels, only to leave you crashing and hungrier than before.

Beware of 'low-fat' or 'diet' labels. These products often replace fat with sugar to improve taste, leading to higher calorie content and minimal nutritional benefit. Always read the labels – if sugar (or one of its many aliases like corn syrup, fructose, etc.) is high on the list, put it back on the shelf.

Also, size matters – avoid mega-sized bags or multi-packs that encourage mindless eating. It's easy to keep reaching into a large bag of snacks without realizing how much you've actually eaten. Whenever possible, portion out your snacks into small containers or buy single-serving packets.

In summary, smart snacking isn't just about choosing the right types of snacks; it's about incorporating them into your day in a way that balances your overall energy and nutrition needs. By selecting whole, unprocessed foods and being mindful about timing and portion sizes, you can enjoy tasty snacks without guilt and keep your health and energy levels on track.

RECAP AND ACTION ITEMS ON THE 9 NUTRITION KNOW-HOW HACKS

By now, you've equipped yourself with a robust toolkit to elevate your nutrition game. Understanding the fundamentals of balanced eating, recognizing the might of superfoods, and mastering the art of smart snacking are pivotal steps towards a healthier, more vibrant you. Let's consolidate what you've learned and transform these insights into actionable steps to seamlessly integrate into your daily life.

Firstly, embrace the basics of macronutrients and micronutrients. Remember, your plate should be a mosaic of nutrients. Aim to include a variety of proteins, carbohydrates, and fats in every meal, and don't forget those vital vitamins and minerals. This balance is key to fueling your body and mind optimally.

Next, become a savvy shopper. Use your new skills in reading food labels to dodge marketing traps and choose foods that offer genuine nutritional value. This means looking beyond flashy labels and understanding what the list of ingredients and nutritional facts actually tells you about the food you're buying. Make this a habit every time you shop.

Portion control is your secret weapon. It's not just what you eat, but how much. Familiarize yourself with serving sizes, use smaller plates, and listen to your body's hunger cues. This will help prevent overeating and maintain energy levels throughout the day.

Harness the power of superfoods. Integrate berries, nuts, seeds, and green leafy vegetables into your diet. These aren't just food; they're fuel and protection for your body. Each superfood packs a unique punch, offering everything from antioxidants to heart-healthy fats.

Finally, snack smart. Keep healthy snack options within reach and time your snacks to avoid energy dips and overeating at meals. Choose snacks that satisfy both your taste buds and your nutritional needs. Avoid snacks that are high in sugar and empty calories, which can sabotage your energy and health goals.

Your journey towards a healthier lifestyle doesn't end here. Each day presents a new opportunity to make choices that benefit your body and mind. Start small, be consistent, and gradually incorporate these practices into your life. Remember, the goal is not just to live longer but to live better.

8

MINDFULNESS AND INNER PEACE

"The real meditation is how you live your life." - *Jon Kabat-Zinn*

Basics of Mindfulness

HACK 64- What is Mindfulness?

Imagine you're sipping your morning cup of tea. Instead of scrolling through your phone, worrying about the day's tasks, you focus solely on the present moment. You notice the steam swirling above the mug, the warmth radiating into your palms, the rich aroma of the tea, and the calmness enveloping your morning. This, in its simplest form, is mindfulness.

Mindfulness is the art of being present and fully engaged with whatever we're doing at the moment — free from distraction or judgement. By bringing your attention to the here and now, mindfulness liberates you from the noise of chaotic thoughts and unnecessary stress. It's about noticing the world around you and finding joy in the mundane.

HACK 65- Everyday Mindfulness Practices

Integrating mindfulness into your daily life doesn't require sitting in silence for long hours. Here are some practical strategies to cultivate mindfulness amidst your busy schedule:

Mindful Breathing:

This can be as simple as taking a few moments to observe your breath. Focus on inhaling deeply through your nose, feeling your chest and belly rise, and then exhaling slowly through your mouth. This practice can be done anywhere — while waiting in line, sitting in traffic, or even during tense moments at work.

Mindful Observation:

Choose a natural object from your immediate environment and focus on watching it for a minute or two. This could be a flower, an insect, or just a patch of sky. Look at it as if you are seeing it for the first time. Notice the colors, shapes, textures, and movement. Engage with it without attaching labels or judgements.

Mindful Listening:

This involves listening to the sounds around you without judgement. It could be the chirping of birds, the hum of a refrigerator, or the distant chatter of people. Listen with curiosity and notice the layers of sounds you typically ignore. This can help you tune into the present moment quickly.

HACK 66- Mindful Eating

Mindful eating is about using mindfulness to reach a state of full attention to your experiences, cravings, and physical cues when eating. Fundamentally, it involves:

Eating slowly and without distraction:

Sit down to eat and invest your full attention in the meal. Avoid distractions like TV or smartphones. By eating slowly, you can savor each bite and better recognize your body's hunger and fullness signals.

Engaging your senses:

Notice the color, texture, aroma, and even the sounds different foods make as you eat them. How do the flavors change with each bite? How does the texture feel in your mouth?

Acknowledging your response to food:

Pay attention to the physical and emotional signals that food elicits. Some foods might make you feel energized, while others can make you feel drowsy.

Appreciating your food:

Think about the effort that went into preparing your meal. Consider the ingredients, the origins of the food, and the effort of the farmers, chefs, and others who brought the meal to your table. This can increase your gratitude and satisfaction with your food.

Integrating mindfulness into your eating habits can transform your relationship with food. It turns eating into a health-generating process, rather than just a mundane activity or, worse, a ground for mindless overeating.

Adopting these practices doesn't require monumental changes. It's about weaving moments of awareness into your day until they become a natural part of your life. Mindfulness is not about getting rid of thoughts; it's about understanding how to live in harmony with them. Start small, be patient with yourself, and observe the subtle shifts in your mood, stress levels, and overall wellness as you engage more deeply with the present moment.

Meditation Made Simple

If you've ever thought that meditation requires you to sit cross-legged for hours, think again. Meditation can be simple, practical, and easily integrated into your everyday routine. Let's demystify it and make it as user-friendly as possible.

HACK 67- Guided Meditation

Starting with guided meditations is like having a personal meditation coach. It's perfect if you find it difficult to know where to begin or if you struggle to focus. Guided meditations walk you through the process and help you find calm and clarity, all without needing to become a Zen master overnight.

To get started, find a quiet space where you won't be disturbed. This could be a corner of your bedroom, a dedicated meditation area, or even a peaceful outdoor spot. Use headphones if you're in a shared space; this helps block out external noise and enhances your focus.

You can access guided meditations through various apps on your smartphone or online. Platforms like Insight Timer, Headspace, and Calm offer a range of guided sessions, from five minutes to an hour, tailored to different aspects of life, whether it's reducing stress, managing anxiety, or even improving sleep.

Choose a session that resonates with what you need. If you're new, start with a short 5 to 10-minute meditation. This could focus on breathing or a body scan, which are great for beginners. As you listen, the guide will prompt you to focus on your breath or notice sensations in your body, helping you to anchor your mind in the present moment.

One key to success with guided meditation is consistency. Try to incorporate it into your daily routine. Perhaps it becomes part of your morning routine, or a way to wind down before bed.

The more regularly you practice, the more natural it will feel, and the deeper the benefits will be.

HACK 68- Breathing Meditations

One of the most powerful, yet simple meditation techniques is focusing on your breath. Breathing meditations can be done anywhere, anytime, making them incredibly versatile and accessible.

To practice a basic breathing meditation, start by finding a comfortable position. You can sit in a chair with your feet flat on the floor, sit on a cushion on the floor with your legs crossed, or even lie down if that's more comfortable.

Close your eyes and take a few deep breaths to settle yourself. Then, let your breath return to its natural rhythm. Pay attention to the sensation of the air entering and leaving your nostrils, or the rise and fall of your chest or abdomen. When your mind wanders, and trust me, it will, gently bring your focus back to your breath. This isn't about stopping thoughts but rather noticing them without attachment and returning to your breathing.

Try this for just five minutes initially. You can use a timer with a gentle sound to signal when the time is up. Over time, as this practice becomes more familiar, you can gradually extend the duration.

Breathing meditations are particularly useful in stressful situations. If you find yourself feeling overwhelmed at work or in any other setting, taking a few minutes to focus solely on your breath can provide a quick reset for your mental state.

HACK 69- Meditative Walking

Meditative walking is a form of meditation in action. Instead of sitting still, it involves walking slowly and mindfully, ideally in a peaceful setting like a park or along a quiet path. This type of meditation is perfect if you find sitting still challenging or if you simply prefer to be more active.

Begin by choosing a quiet place where you can walk back and forth undisturbed for about 10 to 20 feet. Start walking slowly, placing your entire foot on the ground from heel to toe with each step. Focus your attention on the movement of your legs and feet, noticing the sensations as each foot touches and leaves the ground.

Coordinate your breathing with your steps, if possible. For example, you might inhale for three steps and exhale for three steps. Keep your gaze softly focused a few feet ahead to avoid distractions and maintain balance.

Meditative walking is not only about the physical act of walking but also about being aware of your environment. Notice the air on your skin, the sounds around you, and the colors and shapes you see. This helps you connect more deeply with the present moment and can be incredibly grounding.

You can practice meditative walking for as little as ten minutes to feel its calming effects. It's a particularly good way to break up a long day at the office or to clear your mind before making an important decision.

Bringing It All Together

Each of these meditation practices offers a unique way to ease into the world of mindfulness. Whether you choose guided meditations, focus on your breath, or incorporate meditative walking into your day, the key is to find what works best for you and make it a part of your regular routine. Meditation doesn't need to be complicated to be effective. Simple, consistent practice is the most surefire way to experience its many benefits.

Gratitude and Positivity

HACK 70- Keeping a Gratitude Journal

Are you ready to transform your daily life? Let's start with a simple yet profoundly impactful practice: maintaining a gratitude journal. This isn't about jotting down niceties; it's about rewiring your brain to focus on the positive, enhancing your mental health, and, by extension, your overall well-being.

Start by choosing a journal. It doesn't have to be anything fancy — a simple notebook will do. The key is to commit to writing in it regularly. Every night, take a few minutes to reflect on your day and write down three things that you were grateful for. These can be as monumental as a major personal achievement or as simple as the taste of a perfectly brewed morning coffee.

The magic lies in the consistency of the practice. Over time, you'll find that you start looking for things to be grateful for throughout the day, just so you have something to write about. This shift in focus can lead to a more positive outlook on life and a greater appreciation for the little things that often go unnoticed.

What's truly fascinating is the science behind this practice. Studies have shown that maintaining a gratitude journal can lead to greater levels of happiness, reduce depression, and even improve sleep. It's like a natural antidepressant that also boosts your immune system.

HACK 71- Positive Affirmations

Now, let's harness the power of words to shape your reality. Positive affirmations are short, powerful statements that, when repeated often, can influence your subconscious mind, boost your confidence, and reinforce your self-belief.

The key to crafting effective affirmations is to keep them positive, in the present tense, and devoid of any negative words.

For example, instead of saying "I will not worry today," reframe it to "I am filled with peace and calm." The focus is on what you want to feel or achieve, not on what you wish to avoid.

Start your day by stating your affirmations aloud, perhaps while looking in the mirror. Some people find it helpful to write them down and place them where they can always see them—like on a bathroom mirror or the dashboard of their car.

Remember, the goal here is to shift your mental dialogue from self-doubt and fear to confidence and action. It might feel a bit awkward or forced at first, but with regular practice, these affirmations can become a natural part of your thought process, leading to lasting changes in your attitudes and behaviors.

HACK 72- Acts of Kindness

Last but certainly not least, let's talk about the profound impact of acts of kindness. Not only do these actions benefit the recipient, but they also offer incredible advantages to the giver, including increased happiness and a profound sense of connection to others.

Start small. Acts of kindness don't have to be grand gestures. A simple compliment, offering your seat on public transport, or even a smile can make a difference in someone's day. The beauty of kindness is that it's contagious: your actions not only improve the lives of others but can also inspire them to pass on the kindness.

To integrate this practice into your life, aim to perform at least one act of kindness each day. It could be something planned, like volunteering at a local charity, or spontaneous, like paying for the coffee of the person behind you in the queue.

The benefits of this practice are backed by research. Acts of kindness are shown to boost serotonin and dopamine in your brain, which are neurotransmitters that give you feelings of satisfaction and well-being. This biological response has been aptly named the "helper's high."

Incorporating gratitude and positivity into your life isn't just about feeling good. It's about creating a sustainable practice that enhances your mental health, enriches your relationships, and allows you to lead a more fulfilled life. Through gratitude journals, positive affirmations, and acts of kindness, you are setting the groundwork for a life that not only feels good but also adds good to the world.

Remember, the journey to a more positive life starts with a single step. Whether it's scribbling down what you're grateful for, affirming your worth, or extending kindness, each action is a building block towards a happier, healthier you. Embrace these practices, and watch how they transform not just your day, but your entire perspective on life.

RECAP AND ACTION ITEMS ON THE 9 MINDFULNESS AND INNER PEACE HACKS

Congratulations on completing this insightful journey into the realms of Mindfulness and Inner Peace. By now, you've equipped yourself with the fundamental understanding of mindfulness, explored various meditation techniques, and discovered the uplifting power of gratitude and positivity. Let's ensure that these new insights are not just fleeting knowledge, but stepping stones to a more peaceful and fulfilling life.

Practice Daily Mindfulness:

Begin by integrating mindfulness into your daily routine. Set a reminder each morning to take five minutes to focus solely on your breathing—observe the rise and fall of your chest, the sensation of air filling your lungs, and the sounds around you. This simple practice will help you cultivate a habit of being present throughout your day.

Mindful Eating:

Make your next meal an exercise in mindfulness. Turn off all distractions like TV or smartphones, and focus on the flavors, textures, and smells of your food. Eat slowly, savor each bite, and listen to your body's hunger cues. This not only enhances your eating experience but can also lead to better digestion and satisfaction with smaller portions.

Incorporate Mini-Meditations:

Use the guided and breathing meditations you've learnt to refocus during the day. A three-minute breathing exercise can reset your stress levels and boost your focus. Try to schedule these mini-meditations, especially during transitions between different parts of your day.

Go for Meditative Walks:

Choose a natural setting for a walk, where you can practice walking meditation at least once a week. Concentrate on the movement of your legs and feet, the touch of the ground beneath, and the sounds in the environment. This not only enhances your physical health but also connects you deeper with the surroundings.

Gratitude Journal:

Every night, jot down three things you were grateful for that day. They could be as simple as a delicious lunch, a kind gesture from a stranger, or simply the quiet at the end of the day. This practice can significantly shift your mindset over time, leading to greater contentment and positivity.

Positive Affirmations:

Begin your day by stating positive affirmations that resonate with your life goals and values. Phrases like "I am content and calm" or "I choose to make positive healthy choices for myself" can set a positive tone for the day.

Perform Random Acts of Kindness:

Once a week, commit to performing at least one random act of kindness. Whether it's helping a neighbor, donating to a charity, or just giving a compliment, these small acts of kindness can boost your mood and contribute to a more positive outlook on life.

Remember, the transition to a more mindful and peaceful life doesn't happen overnight. It requires commitment and consistent practice. But with each step, you'll find yourself becoming more attuned to the joys of the present moment and more resilient against the chaos of everyday life. Embrace this journey, and watch how it transforms not just your mind, but your health, your energy, and your entire life.

9

BUILDING RESILIENCE

"Do not judge me by my success, judge me by how many times I fell down and got back up again." - Nelson Mandela

Emotional Resilience

HACK 73- Understanding Emotions

First off, let's unpack the suitcase of emotions. You know the drill: joy, sadness, anger, surprise – these guys are just the tip of the iceberg. But what's beneath the surface? Your emotions are not just random feelings; they're complex signals your body sends in response to your surroundings. Think of them as your internal compass, guiding you through life's ups and downs.

To build emotional resilience, start by recognizing and naming your emotions. This might sound simple, but in the heat of the moment, identifying whether you're feeling irritated or downright angry can make a big difference in how you handle the situation. Practice mindfulness; this isn't just a buzzword but a way to tune in to your current emotional state. Mindful breathing exercises or keeping a journal can help you become more aware of your emotional triggers and patterns. Remember, the goal isn't to suppress your feelings but to understand them better.

HACK 74- Coping Mechanisms

Now, understanding your emotions is one thing, but managing them? That's where coping mechanisms come into play. Coping mechanisms are the strategies you use to deal with tricky situations and emotional stress. These can be adaptive or maladaptive, so it's crucial to develop practices that are beneficial rather than those that can lead to more stress or even harm.

Let's talk about some effective strategies. Firstly, there's reframing. This technique involves changing your perspective on a stressful situation. For instance, instead of thinking, "I can't handle this," try, "This is a challenge, but I can work through it." It's about turning a potentially negative experience into an opportunity for growth.

Another resilient strategy is to practice relaxation techniques. These can range from deep breathing and meditation to engaging in yoga or even taking a long walk. The aim is to activate your body's natural relaxation response, which helps reduce stress.

Lastly, don't underestimate the power of humor. Finding something to laugh about can diffuse tension and help you see situations in a new light. It's not about ignoring your problems but giving yourself a moment to reset and gain a fresh perspective.

HACK 75- Seeking Support

A crucial, yet sometimes overlooked aspect of emotional resilience is seeking support. No man is an island, and you don't have to weather the storm alone. Building a support network is key. This could be friends, family, colleagues, or even professional help like therapists or counsellors.

Why is this important? Sharing your thoughts and emotions can help lighten your emotional load and provide you with different viewpoints and strategies to handle your challenges. Moreover, others can offer encouragement, empathy, and validation, which are all essential nutrients for your emotional strength.

Remember, seeking support is not a sign of weakness; it's a strategy of the wise. It's about harnessing the strength and wisdom of others to bolster your own resilience. So, reach out, connect, and cultivate meaningful relationships. They can be your lifeline during tough times.

Building emotional resilience is not an overnight process, but with consistent practice and patience, you can enhance your ability to navigate through life's challenges. Understand your emotions, develop healthy coping mechanisms, and don't shy away from seeking support. By integrating these practices into your life, you're not just surviving; you're thriving.

Physical Resilience

HACK 76- Importance of Regular Check-Ups

Picture this: you're a car. Not just any car, but a finely tuned, high-performance machine that's expected to run smoothly day in and day out. Just like a car requires regular maintenance to avoid breakdowns, your body needs consistent medical check-ups to prevent disease and maintain peak performance. It's easy to skip these appointments when you're feeling fine, but regular check-ups are not just about fixing what's broken; they're about keeping you from breaking in the first place.

Think of your GP as your personal mechanic. An annual physical examination is your opportunity to catch potential health issues before they become serious. It's not just about getting your heart rate checked or stepping onto a scale. It's about establishing a health baseline that can be monitored over time for any significant deviations that might indicate underlying issues.

Your doctor can also tailor these check-ups based on your family history, lifestyle, and age. They might recommend specific screenings such as cholesterol levels, blood pressure measurements, cancer screenings, and more. These proactive measures are crucial because many serious conditions don't have vivid symptoms in the early stages when they're most treatable.

HACK 77- Preventative Measures

Moving on from regular check-ups, let's talk about preventative measures. These are the daily, weekly, or monthly routines that fortify your body's defenses and equip you with the armor to combat the stresses and strains of life.

First off, let's talk diet. Nutrition plays a colossal role in building physical resilience. Foods rich in vitamins, minerals, and antioxidants can boost your immune system, reduce inflammation, and protect your body against disease. Incorporate a variety of fruits, vegetables, lean proteins, and whole grains into your diet. Think of eating a rainbow; the more colors on your plate, the broader the range of nutrients.

Exercise is another pillar of preventative care. Regular physical activity strengthens your heart, muscles, and bones. It enhances your respiratory and immune function, which is essential for warding off illnesses. Moreover, exercise isn't just a preventative tool; it also serves as a therapeutic measure. It can help you manage symptoms of various conditions, from depression to diabetes, and even arthritis.

Sleep must not be overlooked. It's the ultimate repair shop for your body. During sleep, your body heals damaged cells, boosts your immune system, consolidates memories, and recovers from the day's activities. Lack of sleep can lead to a higher susceptibility to illness, not to mention mood swings, impaired cognitive function, and poor energy levels. Aim for 7-9 hours per night to allow your body to perform these vital functions.

HACK 78- Recovery Techniques

Finally, let's delve into recovery techniques. These are crucial for maintaining physical resilience, especially if you're someone who likes to push their limits through exercise or has a demanding daily schedule.

One of the most effective recovery methods is hydration. Water facilitates the transport of nutrients and oxygen to your cells, helps digest food, and maintains body temperature. After any form of intense physical activity, rehydrating helps recover the fluids lost through sweat and can prevent dehydration.

Stretching is another key component of any recovery regime. It helps maintain flexibility, improves your range of motion, and reduces the risk of injuries. Post-exercise stretching can also aid in alleviating muscle tightness and soreness. Incorporate both dynamic stretches as part of your warm-up and static stretches in your cool-down routine.

Mind-body relaxation techniques such as yoga, meditation, and tai chi can also enhance your physical resilience. These practices not only help in physical recovery but also contribute to mental calmness and emotional stability. They teach you to tune into your body's needs and recognize signs of stress and fatigue early on.

Then there's the role of active recovery. This could be a light walk, a gentle swim, or a slow bike ride. Active recovery helps in maintaining a flow of blood and nutrients to the muscles, which can help reduce muscle soreness and speed up the healing process.

Building physical resilience is an ongoing process that requires you to be proactive about your health. Regular check-ups, preventative measures, and proper recovery techniques are all part of a larger strategy aimed at keeping your body's engine running smoothly. By incorporating these practices into your routine, you empower yourself with the tools necessary for a healthier, more energetic life. Remember, the goal isn't just to survive; it's to thrive.

Cognitive Resilience

HACK 79- Brain Exercises

The brain, much like any other part of your body, requires regular workouts to maintain its health and enhance its performance. Engaging in brain exercises can significantly boost your cognitive resilience, allowing you to handle daily stressors with ease and maintain mental clarity. Let's explore some effective brain exercises you might not have considered, which can seamlessly integrate into your daily routine.

First up, puzzles. Not just any puzzles, but specifically crossword puzzles and Sudoku. These aren't just leisure activities; they challenge your brain to think critically and make complex connections, enhancing problem-solving skills and attention to detail. Setting aside just 15 minutes each morning to tackle a Sudoku or crossword puzzle can activate your neural pathways, keeping your mind sharp and ready for the day's challenges.

Next, let's talk about brain training apps. These apps are designed to adapt to your personal cognitive abilities, pushing you just enough to improve but not so much that you're overwhelmed. Apps like Lumosity or Peak offer games that improve various aspects of cognitive functions, including memory, attention, flexibility, speed of processing, and problem-solving skills. By dedicating a few minutes each day to these apps, you can significantly enhance your mental agility.

Lastly, don't underestimate the power of learning a new skill. Whether it's a musical instrument, a new language, or even coding, engaging in learning something new generates new neural connections and boosts brain elasticity. This not only improves cognitive abilities but also equips you with skills that can be both personally fulfilling and professionally beneficial.

HACK 80- Continuous Learning

Continuous learning is the key to keeping your mind engaged and your cognitive abilities sharp. By constantly exposing yourself to new information and experiences, you can forge new neural pathways and reinforce existing ones, enhancing your brain's resilience and capacity to adapt to new challenges.

One of the most accessible ways to engage in continuous learning is through reading. Whether it's non-fiction books that challenge your understanding of the world or fiction that enhances your empathy and creative thinking, reading is a fantastic way to broaden your horizons. Aim to read something every day, even if it's just a few pages. To make this habit stick, choose topics that you're passionate about or curious to explore further.

Another avenue for continuous learning is online courses. Platforms like Coursera, Udemy, and Khan Academy offer courses on nearly every topic imaginable, from psychology and history to technology and business. Many of these courses are free or offer significant knowledge at minimal cost. Dedicating just an hour a week to a new course can dramatically enhance your knowledge base and cognitive capacity.

Lastly, engage in discussions or debates on topics that interest you. This could be through community groups, online forums, or social gatherings. Engaging with diverse perspectives forces you to think critically and articulate your thoughts clearly, sharpening your cognitive abilities and helping you to think on your feet.

HACK 81- Memory Enhancement Techniques

Enhancing your memory is crucial for building cognitive resilience. A strong memory not only aids in learning new skills and knowledge more efficiently but also helps in managing daily tasks and challenges more effectively.

A powerful technique for memory enhancement is the method of loci, also known as the memory palace technique. This method involves visualizing a familiar place and associating each item you want to remember with a specific location within this place. For example, if you need to remember a shopping list, imagine placing each item in different rooms of your house. This technique leverages your spatial memory and makes recall easier and more effective.

Another technique to boost your memory is the practice of chunking. This involves breaking down information into smaller, manageable units, making it easier to process and remember. For instance, if you're trying to memorize a long string of numbers, group them into chunks rather than trying to remember each number individually. This is similar to how you might find it easier to remember a phone number by breaking it into chunks rather than a continuous sequence of digits.

Lastly, regular revision is key to memory retention. The more frequently you review information, the better your brain is at retaining it. Try to revisit important information a few hours after you first learn it, then again a few days later, and periodically after that. This spaced repetition is crucial for moving information from your short-term to long-term memory, solidifying your knowledge base.

By incorporating these strategies into your daily life, you can significantly boost your cognitive resilience, ensuring that your mind remains sharp and efficient. Whether it's through brain exercises, continuous learning, or memory enhancement techniques, each step you take will contribute to a healthier, more resilient cognitive function. Engage regularly and watch as your capacity to handle life's challenges grows, keeping you mentally fit and agile for years to come.

RECAP AND ACTION ITEMS ON THE 9 BUILDING RESILIENCE HACKS

Congratulations on navigating through the essentials of resilience! By dissecting the nuances of emotional, physical, and cognitive resilience, you're now armed with a toolkit that's designed to boost your overall well-being. Let's put that knowledge into action.

Starting with emotional resilience, understanding your emotions is the first step, but action is where change happens. This week, practice mindfulness for 10 minutes each day. Use an app if it helps, or simply sit quietly and observe your thoughts and feelings without judgement. Make a note in your journal about how different emotions surface and subside. This will help you become more aware and in control of your emotional responses.

Next, integrate coping mechanisms into your daily routine. Identify stress triggers and consciously apply positive coping strategies like deep breathing, walking, or talking to a friend when you feel overwhelmed. Establishing these habits now can help you manage stress more effectively in the long run.

For seeking support, don't hesitate to lean on your network. This could be scheduling regular check-ins with a mentor, joining a support group, or even just having coffee with friends who uplift you. Remember, resilience is not about going it alone.

Moving to physical resilience, make that appointment for a regular check-up you've been postponing. It's crucial not only for catching potential health issues early but also for giving you peace of mind.

In terms of preventative measures, adjust one aspect of your lifestyle that could lead to better physical health. Perhaps swap out that late-night snack with something healthier, or try adding a 30-minute walk to your daily routine.

For recovery, if you're sore from your new walking habit, look into techniques such as stretching, warm baths, or even yoga to help your body recover and strengthen.

Lastly, for cognitive resilience, start with brain exercises. Dedicate time each day for puzzles, reading, or other mental challenges. Try to learn something new every week, whether it's a fact, a skill, or a hobby. This not only enhances your brain's ability but keeps life exciting and fulfilling.

Continuous learning can be as simple as listening to a podcast on a topic you know nothing about, or signing up for an online course that piques your interest. Keep your brain engaged and always exploring.

And don't forget about memory enhancement techniques. Implement mnemonic devices for remembering new information or try apps specifically designed to boost memory. Consistent practice is key to improvement.

By embedding these practices into your lifestyle, you will enhance your resilience and enjoy a more vibrant, energetic, and fulfilling life. Remember, resilience is a muscle that strengthens with use. So, get started, keep going, and watch how your life transforms.

10

LIFELONG HABITS FOR HEALTH

"We are what we repeatedly do. Excellence, then, is not an act, but a habit." - Aristotle

Routine Building

HACK 82- Creating Lasting Habits

Let's kick things off with a universal truth: habits shape our lives. Whether you're a CEO, a stay-at-home parent, or a freelance artist, your daily habits are the invisible architecture of your everyday existence. But here's the kicker: building habits that stick is less about willpower and more about strategy.

The first step in creating lasting habits is to understand the psychology behind habit formation. The renowned model introduced by Charles Duhigg, which consists of a cue, a routine, and a reward, provides a fantastic blueprint. Let's break this down:

Cue:

Identify a consistent trigger that tells your brain to go into automatic mode. This could be as simple as placing your running shoes next to your bed, so you see them first thing in the morning

Routine:

This is the behavior itself, the action you want to turn into a habit. For instance, it might be going for a run

Reward:

This is something that your brain likes that helps it remember the "habit loop" in the future. Maybe it's the endorphin rush after a run, or perhaps you treat yourself to a delicious smoothie afterwards.

To make a habit stick, it needs to fit into your life. This means setting achievable goals. If you aim to meditate daily, start with just five minutes rather than thirty. Small steps are not just easier; they're more sustainable.

HACK 83- Morning Routines

Morning routines are often heralded as the secret weapon of the highly successful. Why? Because they set the tone for the rest of the day. A solid morning routine can boost your energy levels, sharpen your focus, and increase your productivity.

So, how do you craft a morning routine that catapults you into a day of success? Start by considering what energizes you. For some, it's a vigorous 20-minute workout; for others, it might be quietly sipping coffee while journaling.

Here's a simple structure to get you started:-

Wake up at the same time every day:

Yes, even on weekends. This helps regulate your body's internal clock and improves your sleep quality over time

Hydrate:

Drink a glass of water first thing. Overnight, you become dehydrated, so this is crucial

Move:

Whether it's yoga, stretching, or a full-blown gym session, get your body moving. It wakes up your mind and body

Meditate:

Just a few minutes can help clear your mind and reduce stress

Plan:

Take a moment to look at your tasks for the day. Prioritizing early can help you stay organized and focused.

Remember, your morning routine should fit who you are. If meditation isn't your thing, maybe reading or listening to a podcast is. The key is consistency and finding what genuinely works for you.

HACK 84- Evening Routines

Just as a morning routine sets the stage for the day, an evening routine can help you wind down and ensure a good night's sleep — critical for recovery and performance.

Developing an effective evening routine starts with unplugging. Exposure to blue light from screens can disrupt your sleep cycle, so try to turn off electronic devices at least an hour before bed. Instead, you might:

Read a book:

This can help ease the transition between wakefulness and sleep

Reflect:

Spend a few minutes reflecting on the day. What went well? What could be improved?

Prepare for tomorrow:

Lay out your clothes for the next day or prepare your breakfast. It'll give you a head start.

A key component of a good evening routine is consistency. Going to bed and waking up at the same time each day helps regulate your body's clock and improves your overall sleep quality.

Lastly, try to create a relaxing environment in your bedroom. A cool, dark, and quiet room can significantly enhance the quality of your sleep. Consider using aromatherapy or white noise machines if you find it hard to unwind.

In essence, routine building is all about setting yourself up for success in a way that feels natural and sustainable. Whether it's the energizing thrust of a morning ritual or the calming descent of an evening routine, these structured moments can profoundly impact your health and general well-being. By embedding these practices into your daily life, you're not just surviving; you're thriving.

Technology for Health

In this digital age, where technology intertwines with nearly every aspect of our lives, it's no wonder that it has also become a pivotal ally in managing and enhancing our health. From fitness apps that fit right into your pocket to online resources and the burgeoning field of telemedicine, technology offers tools that can significantly optimize your health management. Let's dive into how you can leverage these innovations to your advantage.

HACK 85- Using Apps for Fitness

Consider your smartphone as a personal trainer, nutritionist, and health monitor all rolled into one. Fitness apps are revolutionizing the way people engage with their health routines. Whether you are a beginner or an avid fitness enthusiast, there is an app tailored to your needs.

For starters, apps like MyFitnessPal help you track your dietary intake and monitor calories, providing a clear picture of your nutritional habits. It's like having a dietary consultant in your pocket, nudging you towards healthier choices every day. Similarly, Strava or Nike Run Club can transform your running routine by tracking your routes, speeds, and providing a platform to compete with friends, adding a fun and interactive element to your workouts.

Moreover, for those who find it challenging to visit a gym

regularly, apps like Freeletics use AI to create personalized bodyweight training routines that you can perform anywhere, anytime. No equipment? No problem. Your living room can now double as your fitness studio.

The key is consistency. Allow these apps to push notifications reminding you of workout times, hydration, and even meditation sessions. These little pings can serve as the gentle nudges you need to make health a daily habit.

HACK 86- Online Health Resources

The internet is a treasure trove of information, and when it comes to health, the wealth of knowledge is vast and varied. Websites like WebMD, Mayo Clinic, and NHS provide credible information that can help you better understand symptoms, diseases, and the necessary preventive measures. These resources are written by professionals and often peer-reviewed, ensuring the information is not only comprehensive but also trustworthy.

However, the trick is to use these resources wisely. It's easy to tumble down the rabbit hole of symptom-checking and self-diagnosis, which can sometimes lead to unnecessary anxiety. Use these sites to educate yourself about possible health conditions but always consult with a healthcare professional for diagnoses and treatment plans.

Furthermore, blogs and forums like Reddit's r/fitness or

r/health can also be useful. They provide a platform for community interaction where you can share experiences, tips, and get support from others who are on similar health journeys. Remember, while these communities can offer support and advice, the authenticity of individual advice can vary, so approach with a critical mind.

HACK 87- Benefits of Telemedicine

Telemedicine, a term that has gained tremendous traction especially in the post-pandemic era, refers to the practice of caring for patients remotely when the provider and patient are not physically present with each other. This technology has proven to be a game changer in making healthcare accessible for everyone.

With telemedicine, routine check-ups, initial consultations, and follow-up visits can be conducted via video calls, thus saving you time and the hassle of commuting. This is particularly beneficial if you live in a remote area or have mobility challenges. Platforms like Babylon Health and Push Doctor provide these services at your convenience, ensuring that healthcare fits into your busy schedule rather than disrupting it.

Telemedicine also extends to mental health. Platforms like Talkspace and BetterHelp offer counselling services through text, voice, and video calls, making mental health support more accessible and less stigmatized. It's like having a therapist in your pocket, available at a moment's notice.

Moreover, telemedicine can facilitate better health monitoring. For patients with chronic conditions like diabetes or hypertension, apps can help track your vitals and share them directly with your doctor in real-time, enabling timely interventions and adjustments to treatments.

Incorporating technology into your health regimen isn't just about staying with the trends; it's about actively choosing tools and resources that enhance your ability to live a healthier, more fulfilled life. By harnessing the power of apps, online resources, and telemedicine, you're setting up a framework that supports your health goals in a modern, efficient, and interactive way. Whether it's improving your physical fitness, gaining knowledge, or accessing healthcare professionals from the comfort of your home, technology offers myriad possibilities to keep you on the path to wellness.

Community and Connection

HACK 88- Joining Health Groups

Ever found yourself needing a little push to lace up those trainers or swap that cheeky slice of cake for a crisp apple? You're not alone. That's where the magic of health groups comes in. Imagine a powerhouse of motivation and support, all geared towards helping you stick to your health goals. Now, that's a game changer.

Joining a health group isn't just about having company during workouts; it's about surrounding yourself with a community that shares your aspirations and challenges. These groups vary from running clubs and yoga classes to online forums focused on nutrition and mental wellbeing. What's fantastic is that there's something for everyone. Whether you're a beginner or a seasoned fitness enthusiast, finding a group that resonates with your needs and personality can significantly amplify your commitment to a healthier lifestyle.

Let's talk about the ripple effect of joining these groups. Firstly, the social commitment. Announcing your goals in a group sets a powerful psychological mechanism into motion – you're less likely to hit snooze on your alarm when you know your buddy is waiting for you in the cold for that morning run. Secondly, learning from peers. There's always someone who's been where you are, and their knowledge and experience can steer you away from common pitfalls, enhancing your journey towards better health.

Moreover, these groups often organize events and challenges, which can add a fun and competitive element to your routine. Whether it's a 5K run, a yoga challenge, or a month without sugar, these activities can keep your motivation high and make your health journey enjoyable.

HACK 89 - Volunteering

Now, how about combining the joy of helping others with your pursuit of health? Volunteering offers this unique blend. Engaging in community service is not only soul-enriching but also surprisingly beneficial for your physical health and mental resilience. Whether it's helping out at a local food bank, coaching a little league team, or participating in community clean-ups, the act of giving back carries rich rewards.

The physical activity involved in most volunteer work can contribute significantly to your fitness. Think about it - gardening in the community park, walking dogs for a local animal shelter, or setting up a charity event. These activities get you moving, almost like stealth exercise, packed within meaningful tasks.

Then there's the mental health aspect. Volunteering is known to reduce stress, combat depression, and provide a profound sense of purpose. When you focus on meeting the needs of others, the chronic stressors of daily life can seem to diminish, and the social interaction helps buffer loneliness and anxiety.

Lastly, let's not forget the broader health implications. Studies have shown that those who volunteer have a lower mortality rate than those who do not, even when considering factors like physical health. This could be due to the combination of increased physical activity, social interaction, and the psychological benefits of altruism.

HACK 90- Family Health Initiatives

Bringing health into the family circle can transform an individual quest into a thrilling group adventure. When families engage together in health initiatives, every member wins. This could be as simple as planning a weekly menu with balanced meals, organizing family sports days, or setting collective health goals like reducing screen time.

The beauty of family health initiatives lies in their ability to teach younger family members about healthy living from an early age. Kids who see their parents prioritizing health are more likely to adopt these habits themselves. This can set the foundation for a lifetime of healthy choices, not to mention the immediate benefits like better concentration in school and improved emotional wellbeing.

Moreover, when you tackle health as a family, it becomes easier to stay on track. There's an in-built support system where everyone encourages each other. If one member struggles, the family can rally to support them, ensuring that no one is left behind. This can be particularly effective in overcoming challenges such as quitting smoking or cutting down on junk food.

Additionally, family health initiatives can be a lot of fun, bringing a sense of play into what might otherwise be a chore. Whether it's a dance-off in the living room, a weekend hike, or preparing a new recipe together, these activities strengthen familial bonds and create joyful memories, all while improving health.

In conclusion, weaving the threads of community, volunteering, and family into the fabric of your health journey does more than just ensure a robust support network; it enriches your life, making the path to health a shared and joyous journey. So why not take that step today? Your body, mind, and community will thank you for it.

RECAP AND ACTION ITEMS ON THE 9 LIFELONG HABITS FOR HEALTH HACKS

As you've journeyed through the exploration of lifelong habits for health, you've armed yourself with powerful strategies to overhaul your well-being and energy levels. Now, it's time to put these insights into action and truly transform your life.

Firstly, let's talk about routine building. You understand the importance of creating lasting habits. Start by identifying one small health habit you want to develop—maybe it's drinking a glass of water first thing in the morning or taking a ten-minute walk after dinner. Commit to this habit for the next 30 days, marking each successful day on a calendar to visually track your progress.

For your morning routine, consider setting a fixed wake-up time and kick-starting your day with a series of stretches or a short meditation session. This will not only wake up your body but also prep your mind for the day ahead. In the evenings, wind down by disconnecting from electronic devices at least an hour before bed, perhaps replacing screen time with reading a book or planning the next day.

Moving on to technology for health, leverage the power of apps to enhance your fitness and health monitoring. Choose an app that aligns with your fitness goals, be it yoga, running, or strength training, and use it consistently to track your progress and stay motivated. Don't forget to explore online health resources; these can offer valuable tips and personalized advice. Also, consider the benefits of telemedicine for your routine medical consultations, making healthcare more accessible and less time-consuming.

Lastly, never underestimate the power of community and connection. Join a health group or a fitness class that not only helps you stay physically active but also connects you with like-minded individuals. Consider volunteering; giving back to the community can significantly boost your mental health and sense of well-being. And, involve your family in your health initiatives, perhaps planning weekend hikes or cooking healthy meals together, making wellness a shared goal.

Transforming your health is a journey, not a sprint. Take it one step at a time, integrate these practices into your life, and watch as your health, energy, and fulfilment levels soar. Remember, the best time to start is now. Make your health a priority—you deserve it.

11

SOCIAL WELLNESS AND RELATIONSHIPS

"No man is an island, entire of itself; every man is a piece of the continent, a part of the main." – John Donne

Building Strong Connections

In the pursuit of a healthier, more fulfilling life, how often do you consider the role of your social connections? It's not just about eating right or hitting the gym; the relationships you cultivate can significantly impact your well-being. Let's dive into how you can build strong connections that not only enrich your life but could also enhance your health and energy levels.

HACK 91- Nurturing Friendships

Friendships are the spices that flavor our lives. They can provide comfort during tough times, laughter during good times, and insight when we're lost. However, like any worthwhile endeavor, friendships require nurturing to grow and thrive.

Start by taking stock of your current friendships. Which ones leave you feeling positive and energized? These are the friendships to focus on. Life can get incredibly busy, but making time for these relationships is crucial. Schedule regular catch-ups, whether they're face-to-face or virtual. Consistency is key—regular contact helps to keep the bond strong.

Communication is the backbone of any relationship. When catching up with friends, make sure it's a two-way street. Listen intently, but also share your own experiences and feelings. Vulnerability can strengthen bonds, creating deeper, more meaningful connections.

Remember, quality trumps quantity. It's better to have a few close friends you can rely on than a multitude of acquaintances you barely know. Invest in these relationships by celebrating successes, offering support during failures, and being present in each other's lives. Simple acts like remembering birthdays, anniversaries, or even just sending a message to check in can make a significant difference.

HACK 92- Effective Communication Skills

Effective communication is more than just exchanging information; it's about understanding the emotion and intentions behind the information. As you aim to build strong connections, refining your communication skills can be a game changer.

Firstly, practice active listening. This doesn't just mean nodding along while someone talks; it involves really hearing what the other person is saying and showing that you understand. Reflect back what you've heard and ask clarifying questions. This shows that you value what they're saying and are engaged in the conversation.

Be mindful of not just what you say, but how you say it. Tone, timing, and delivery can all affect how your message is received. Aim for clarity and be direct, but also considerate. Avoid misunderstandings by keeping your messages simple and straightforward.

Non-verbal cues are also a huge part of communication. Pay attention to body language, both your own and others'. A lot can be conveyed through eye contact, facial expressions, and posture. These can all indicate how someone really feels, beyond what they're saying.

Conflict is inevitable in any relationship, but don't shy away from it. Handle disagreements with empathy and patience.

Aim to resolve conflicts by understanding the other person's perspective and coming to a mutual solution, rather than winning the argument. This approach not only resolves the immediate issue but also strengthens the relationship long-term.

HACK 93- Expanding Your Social Network

While deepening existing relationships is essential, expanding your social network is equally important. Meeting new people can introduce fresh ideas, perspectives, and opportunities into your life.

One effective way to meet new people is by exploring new interests or hobbies. Join clubs, classes, or groups that align with your interests. This not only puts you in touch with like-minded individuals but also gives you a shared topic to bond over.

Networking events can be goldmines for expanding your social circle. Approach these gatherings with the mindset of 'what can I offer' rather than 'what can I get'. This shift in perspective makes interactions more authentic and builds a foundation for mutual respect and potential friendships.

Don't forget the power of volunteering. This is a fantastic way to meet people while giving back to the community. It's a win-win: you contribute to a cause you care about and connect with others who share your values.

Lastly, leverage technology. Social media and networking platforms are great tools for connecting with others. However, use them wisely. Engage in meaningful conversations and try to transition online connections to in-person meetings when possible.

Building strong connections is an art that entails nurturing existing friendships, honing your communication skills, and expanding your social network. Each step you take towards enhancing these skills not only enriches your social life but also bolsters your overall health and well-being. Remember, the goal is to foster relationships that are not only fulfilling but also supportive and uplifting, creating a network that powers you through life's ups and downs.

Family Dynamics and Wellness

HACK 94- Strengthening Family Bonds

In the bustling rhythm of everyday life, family bonds can sometimes take a back seat to deadlines, social commitments, and personal pursuits. Yet, the strength of your family ties can significantly influence your emotional and physical health. To foster deeper connections with your family members, consider implementing regular family meetings. This isn't just about gathering around the dinner table; it's about creating a structured opportunity where each member can voice their thoughts, feelings, and concerns in a supportive environment. It's about ensuring everyone feels heard and valued.

Setting up a 'no tech' rule during these meetings can enhance attentiveness and presence. In today's digital age, this might feel like a challenge, but the undivided attention boosts the quality of interactions. Furthermore, engaging in activities that all family members enjoy can also reinforce bonds. Whether it's a weekly board game night, a cooking session, or a shared hobby, these activities provide relaxed settings that encourage spontaneous conversations and joyous moments.

Another vital component is the appreciation ritual. It can be as simple as expressing what you appreciate about each other at the end of the day or week. This practice not only uplifts the mood but also helps in building mutual respect and affection, reinforcing the emotional connections within the family.

HACK 95- Managing Family Conflicts

Conflict is a natural part of any relationship, and families are no exception. Managing these conflicts healthily can prevent them from escalating and affecting the overall family dynamics. One effective method is to establish clear communication rules that discourage shouting, interruptions, and any form of disrespect. Encourage a culture where problems are discussed openly rather than swept under the rug. This transparency helps in addressing issues before they grow into larger conflicts.

When a disagreement arises, try to understand the underlying concerns. Often, conflicts stem from unmet needs or miscommunications. By focusing on the needs rather than the surface emotions, you can approach the situation with empathy and find solutions that accommodate everyone's concerns. Moreover, learning to choose your battles wisely is crucial. Not every disagreement needs to be a full-blown conflict; sometimes, letting go of minor irritations can lead to a more peaceful and cooperative environment.

Implementing conflict resolution tools like 'time-outs' can also be beneficial. When emotions run high, taking a break can help everyone cool down and gain perspective. After a pause, discussions can resume with a calmer, more constructive approach that favors resolution over blame.

HACK 96- Supporting Each Other's Health

The well-being of each family member contributes to the health of the entire family unit. Therefore, creating a supportive environment that promotes healthy habits is essential. One effective strategy is to engage in healthy activities together. This might include planning nutritious meals, exercising as a family, or even cultivating a vegetable garden. Such activities not only improve physical health but also provide opportunities for spending quality time together, thereby strengthening emotional bonds.

Mental health is equally important. Encourage open conversations about feelings and challenges. This not only destigmatizes mental health issues but also makes it easier for family members to seek support when needed. Additionally, be proactive in learning about mental health, including recognizing signs of stress or depression. This knowledge can be crucial in providing timely support and understanding.

Lastly, respect individual health journeys. Each family member may have different health needs and goals. Supporting these individual journeys can include accommodating dietary restrictions, recognizing personal space needs, or supporting each other's health appointments and routines. This respect for individual needs reinforces a supportive family environment where everyone feels looked after and valued.

In conclusion, integrating these practices into your family life can transform everyday interactions and significantly enhance the health and happiness of your family unit. By actively working on strengthening bonds, managing conflicts effectively, and supporting each other's health, you lay down the foundation for a dynamic and resilient family environment. Embrace these strategies with openness and consistency, and watch as they bring about profound positive changes in your family dynamics.

Social Well-being in the Community

HACK 97- Community Involvement

In the bustling world we live in, it's easy to get lost in the shuffle of personal and professional commitments. However, stepping outside your immediate circle and engaging with the wider community can profoundly impact your health and overall happiness. When you involve yourself in the community, you're not just giving back – you're also setting the stage for personal growth and building a network of support that can enhance your life in unexpected ways.

Start small. Look for local events that resonate with your interests. Whether it's a community garden, a book club, or a local sports team, participating in these activities can provide a sense of belonging and shared purpose. It's not just about filling your calendar; it's about connecting in meaningful ways that align with your values and interests.

Moreover, community involvement can lead to a deeper understanding of diverse perspectives and challenges within your locality. This heightened awareness can cultivate empathy, a critical component in maintaining strong mental health and fostering relationships. By stepping into different community roles, you might find yourself developing skills you didn't know you had, boosting your confidence and sense of achievement.

Next, consider attending community meetings or joining local boards. This can provide insight into the inner workings of your community and offer opportunities to contribute to decision-making processes that affect your environment. It's empowering to have a say in the changes you want to see, and such involvement can make you feel more connected and responsible for the well-being of your area.

Remember, the key to making the most out of your community involvement is consistency. Regular participation not only helps in building stronger connections but also establishes you as a reliable and committed member of the community. This can open doors to new friendships and professional opportunities that might not have been available otherwise.

HACK 98- Volunteering and Giving Back

Volunteering is one of the most rewarding ways to enrich your life and the lives of others. It's a tangible expression of gratitude and a powerful means to extend your influence beyond your immediate surroundings. When you volunteer, you do more than help others – you also gain experiences that can transform your own outlook and health.

Choose a cause you are passionate about. Whether it's helping at a local food bank, tutoring children, or caring for animals at a shelter, engaging in work that resonates with your heart will make the experience more fulfilling. This passion fuels perseverance, especially when the going gets tough, and the emotional rewards of your efforts mirror the physical and mental energy you invest.

Volunteering can also significantly boost your mental health. It reduces stress, combats depression, and provides a profound sense of purpose. These emotional benefits are critical in maintaining a balanced life and can improve your overall well-being. Moreover, the social aspect of volunteering allows you to meet and connect with like-minded individuals who share your passions and values, which can lead to lasting friendships and a strong sense of community connectedness.

Don't overlook the importance of regular engagement. Consistent volunteering not only helps the organization but also ensures that you remain connected to the cause and the community. It allows you to see the real impact of your contributions over time, enhancing the sense of accomplishment and emotional satisfaction that comes from giving back.

HACK 99- Building Support Networks

In the journey of life, having a robust support network can be your greatest asset. Community isn't just about geographical boundaries; it's about forging connections that provide support and enhance resilience during challenging times. Building these networks within your community can safeguard your mental and emotional health and provide a platform for mutual support.

Start by identifying community spaces that offer support groups or clubs that match your interests or current life challenges. Whether it's a group for new parents, a book discussion club, or a fitness group, such communities can offer both emotional and practical support. Sharing experiences and solutions with people who understand your situation can reduce feelings of isolation and provide diverse perspectives that can help you navigate life's ups and downs.

Furthermore, consider using technology to enhance your community connections. Online forums, social media groups, and community apps can extend your support network beyond physical meetings and provide a platform for continuous connection and support. Whether it's advice, a listening ear, or sharing a success, these digital spaces can be invaluable in maintaining strong ties with your community peers.

Lastly, be proactive in your interactions. While it's essential to seek support when needed, offering support to others can reinforce your role within the network and deepen the bonds of trust and mutual respect. The give-and-take nature of strong support networks not only fosters individual well-being but also strengthens the entire community fabric.

By engaging in community involvement, volunteering, and building robust support networks, you enhance not just your own life but also contribute to the vitality and resilience of your wider community. These actions weave together the social fabric that supports personal and collective well-being, creating a fulfilling and supported life.

RECAP AND ACTION ITEMS ON THE 9 SOCIAL WELLNESS AND RELATIONSHIPS HACKS

Congratulations on powering through this vital chapter on Social Wellness and Relationships. By now, you should have a robust toolkit to not only enhance your personal connections but also to positively impact your family dynamics and engage more deeply with your community.

Let's break down what you've learned into actionable steps that you can start implementing today to see real changes in your life.

Nurture Your Friendships:

Make it a priority to reach out to a friend at least once a week. Whether it's a quick call, a text, or meeting up for coffee, keeping the lines of communication open strengthens bonds. Try setting a reminder on your phone to catch up with someone different each week.

Hone Your Communication Skills:

Effective communication is key in all relationships. Practice active listening in your next conversation. This means fully concentrating on what is being said rather than just passively hearing the message of the speaker. Reflect back what you've heard to ensure understanding and validation.

Expand Your Social Network:

Attend a new club or group meeting in your area that aligns with your interests. This could be anything from a book club to a sports team. Pushing yourself out of your comfort zone can be rewarding and fun.

Strengthen Family Bonds:

Schedule regular family meetings or outings where everyone gets a chance to voice their feelings and thoughts. This could be a weekly dinner where each member shares the highlight of their week.

Manage Family Conflicts:

When disagreements arise, address them calmly and promptly. Use "I" statements to express how you feel without blaming others, which could help in reducing tension and misunderstanding.

Support Each Other's Health:

Initiate a family health challenge, such as daily walks or a cooking contest using healthy recipes. It's a great way to spend time together while encouraging healthy habits.

Get Involved in Your Community:

Look for opportunities where you can contribute, maybe through local councils or charities. Engaging in community planning or improvement projects can give you a sense of belonging and accomplishment.

Volunteer and Give Back:

Choose a cause you care about and volunteer some of your time. This not only aids those in need but can also connect you with like-minded individuals.

Build Support Networks:

Finally, remember you're not alone. Join support groups or networks in your community that resonate with your personal experiences or challenges. These groups provide emotional support and advice crucial for personal growth and well-being.

By integrating these steps into your life, you'll not only improve your health and energy but also deepen the relationships that make life worth living. Remember, the quality of your relationships is the single most significant predictor of happiness. So, take these steps seriously, have fun with them, and watch as your life transforms.

EMBRACING YOUR OPTIMAL SELF

As you turn the final page of this journey, it's essential to pause and reflect on the transformative path you've embarked upon. This isn't merely the end of a book; it's the beginning of a profound personal revolution. The strategies and insights laid out in the preceding chapters are stepping stones towards a more vibrant, fulfilled, and optimized you.

You've been equipped with the knowledge to wake up to wellness, declutter your mind for mental clarity, preemptively tackle stress, and enhance the quality of your sleep. Moreover, the innovative hydration hacks and subsequent strategies introduced have provided a well-rounded toolkit to elevate your daily life. But what comes next is entirely up to you.

Transformation is not a passive process. It doesn't suffice to read about change; change demands action. The true essence of this journey lies in application—the deliberate, consistent application of learned principles. It's about making incremental improvements that collectively amount to significant change. It's about not just doing different but being different.

Consider how each strategy can be integrated into your daily routine. How will you ensure that you wake up each day with a purpose and a passion? What systems will you put in place to maintain mental clarity and keep stress at bay? How will you guard your sleep as fervently as you pursue your waking ambitions? The answers to these questions will sculpt your tomorrow.

Remember, the pursuit of optimization is ongoing and ever-evolving. As you grow and your circumstances change, so too will your needs. This book is a compass, not a map. It points you in the direction of well-being and personal excellence, but the steps you take, the pace you maintain, and the destinations you reach are yours to determine.

Moreover, this journey is not meant to be solitary. The value of a supportive network—a community of like-minded individuals who share your commitment to growth—cannot be overstated. Engage with others who are on similar paths. Share your successes and challenges, learn from each other, and grow together. The collective energy of a community focused on optimization can propel you to heights that might be unreachable alone.

Yet, there are moments in every quest when guidance specific to your unique circumstances is invaluable. Perhaps you'll find yourself facing challenges that require more specialized strategies or you might seek to accelerate your journey with expert advice tailored specifically to your goals. In these moments, professional help can be a powerful catalyst.

If you feel compelled to seek out such expertise, consider reaching out for professional guidance. Whether it's to deepen your understanding of a particular topic discussed in this book or to develop a personalized plan that addresses your unique challenges and aspirations, professional support can transform complexity into clarity and intention into action.

As you move forward, keep the principles of this book at the forefront of your mind. Let them guide your decisions, influence your actions, and shape your future. The path to optimization is rich with opportunity and growth, and every step forward is a step towards becoming the best version of yourselves.

Reflect on what you've learned, but more importantly, act on it. Test theories, adjust strategies, and find what works best for you. This is not the conclusion of your journey but a commencement. A call to action not just to think differently, but to live differently.

Optimization is not a destination but a way of travelling. Embrace it with enthusiasm and commitment, and there is no limit to what you can achieve. The ultimate measure of your journey through this book will not be where you stand now but where you go from here.

Let this closing chapter be a starting bell, ringing you into action, urging you forward towards a life not just lived, but optimized. Embrace the challenge with enthusiasm, and step into your most vibrant, effective, and fulfilling life.

Enjoyed the book?

If this book helped you or brought you some enjoyment, please take a moment to leave a quick review online.

It only takes a minute, but it makes a huge difference to me and helps others discover the book too.

Your feedback means the world and thanks for your support!

www.ingramcontent.com/pod-product-compliance
Lightning Source LLC
Chambersburg PA
CBHW071922210526
45479CB00002B/512